PERSON-CENTRED
DEMENTIA CARE

PERSON-CENTRED DEMENTIA CARE

Making Services Better with the VIPS Framework

Dawn Brooker and Isabelle Latham

Jessica Kingsley *Publishers*
London and Philadelphia

First edition published in 2006
This edition published in 2016
by Jessica Kingsley Publishers
73 Collier Street
London N1 9BE, UK
and
400 Market Street, Suite 400
Philadelphia, PA 19106, USA

www.jkp.com

Library of Congress Cataloging in Publication Data
Brooker, Dawn, 1959- , author.
Person-centred dementia care : making services better with
the VIPS framework / Dawn Brooker and
Isabelle Latham. -- Second edition.
p. ; cm.
Includes bibliographical references and index.
ISBN 978-1-84905-666-3 (alk. paper)
I. Latham, Isabelle, author. II. Title.
[DNLM: 1. Dementia--nursing. 2. Nurse-Patient Relations.
3. Nursing Care. 4. Patient-Centered Care--
methods. WM 220]
RC521
616.8'3--dc23
2015025408

British Library Cataloguing in Publication Data
A CIP catalogue record for this book is available from the British Library

ISBN 978 1 84905 666 3
eISBN 978 1 78450 170 9

Printed and bound in Great Britain

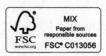

Contents

Acknowledgements

The second edition of this book, like the first, has drawn on lessons learnt from many practitioners, researchers and people whose lives are directly affected by dementia. The first edition's success far outstripped expectations in terms of readership and has been translated into more languages than we have been able to keep track of. Providing best practice in person-centred dementia care is a global challenge that can feel overwhelming. We all have much to learn from each other, whatever our background and whatever country we are from. What people liked about the first edition of *Person Centred Dementia Care – Making Services Better* was that it provided practical and manageable approaches that care providers could use whatever their role. People liked the VIPS structure and the photocopiable resource has also helped with the practical application. We have endeavoured to keep true to these principles within this second edition.

Since writing the first edition, Dawn has set up the Association for Dementia Studies at the University of Worcester in the UK. The ambition, to set up a research centre dedicated to developing evidence-based practical ways of helping people live well with dementia, was realised in 2009. The Association for Dementia Studies now has an active programme of research and education programmes which has touched the lives of thousands of people. Isabelle joined the Association in 2011 following a career in care practice. Initially she worked on the CHOICE research programme. She is now a senior lecturer and leads on a broad range of research and education projects.

The team (past and present) at the Association for Dementia Studies have supported and inspired us all the way in writing this book but special thanks go to Teresa Atkinson, Jen Bray, Mary Bruce, Helen

Cain, Christine Carter, Bernie Coope, Kay De Vries, Carole Edwards, Debbie Fox, Michal Herz, Nicola Jacobson, Karan Jutlla, Jenny La Fontaine, Helen Malbon, David Moore, Guy Page, Wendy Perry, Liz Peel, Sue Pinfold-Brown, Hazel Ratcliffe, Kate Read, Zuleika Sankey and Mike Watts.

In addition we are grateful to our colleagues and supporters in the UK and overseas who have helped us shape our thinking in the past six years: Peter Ashley, Caroline Baker, Clive Ballard, Alistair Burns, Nicky Bradbury, Andy Bradley, Ian Bennett, Linda Clare, Sam Davis, Tom Dening, Murna Downs, Rose-Marie Dröes, David Edvardsson, Knut Engedal, Elena Fernández Gamarra, Simon Foster, Jane Fossey, Carol Fusek, Cathy Greenblat, Marilyn Hartle, June Hennell, LaDonna Jensen, Yun-Hee Jeon, David Jolley, John Killick, Bernie McCarthy, Hazel May, Yutaka Mizuno, Virginia Moore, Esme Moniz-Cook, Wendy Moyle, Yasuko Murata, Michiko Nakagawa, Yuko Nakamura, Keith Oliver, Martin Orrell, Patricia Paquete, Al Power, Anne Marie Mork Rokstad, Janne Rosvik, Justine Schneider, Graham Stokes, Claire Surr, Myrra Vernooij-Dassen, Josep Vila Miravent, Steve Sabat, Philippa Shreeve, Yves Smith-White, Jon Snaedal, Mizue Suzuki, Kate Swaffer and Bob Woods. Cathy Greenblat's photos and Christine Bryden's writing have continued to be both an inspiration and a validation.

We have drawn particularly on our experience of working on two inspiring research programmes in the writing of this book and we are grateful to all our colleagues and funders on both of these. The first is the CHOICE Programme (2010–2012) was led by Anne Killett University of East Anglia in collaboration with Dawn Brooker, Jenny La Fontaine & Isabelle Latham at University of Worcester; Alison Bowes, Fiona Kelly & Mike Wilson at University of Stirling; Martin O'Neill at Cardiff University and Diane Burns at University of Sheffield and included valuable support from Bridget Penhale, Paula Hyde, Fiona Poland, Richard Gray, Nick Jenkins & Heather Strange. We are particularly grateful to the care homes including residents, relatives, visitors and staff who volunteered to take part in the project. This research was funded through the PANICOA programme by the Department of Health and Comic Relief. The views expressed in this book are those of the authors and do not reflect those of the Department of Health or Comic Relief.

The second was the FITS into Practice programme that was led by the Association for Dementia Studies, University of Worcester and funded by the Alzheimer's Society. The project has looked at reducing the prescription of anti-psychotics for people living with dementia in care homes, through person-centred approaches and specific interventions. It followed on from an original randomised controlled trial of the FITS training programme which produced significant results in terms of anti-psychotic reduction developed by King's College London, and Universities of Oxford and Newcastle, and Oxford Health NHS Trust. We are grateful to all who participated in the research.

In particular we are grateful to people living with dementia, their families, the staff and visitors of the many care organisations who have taken part in our research and participated in our education programmes. Your passion and commitment inspire our work.

Dawn Brooker and Isabelle Latham 2015

Part 1
Unpacking Person-centred Care

1

What is Person-centred Care?

Person-centred care is written into policy documents, education courses, mission statements, care-planning tools, job descriptions and protocols in almost every part of the dementia care scene. It seems that any dementia care initiative has to claim to be 'pc' (person-centred) in order to be 'PC' (politically correct). Many of us live with the uneasy knowledge, however, that, although the words sound good, the lived experience of care for people with dementia – particularly for those living in long-term care – is anything but person-centred. As with many terms that are frequently used, there is a tendency for person-centred care to mean different things to different people in different contexts. In our discussions with practitioners, researchers and people with dementia and their families, it is obvious that the concepts in person-centred care are not easy to understand or articulate in a straightforward manner. To some, it means individualised care. To others, it is a value base. There are people who see it as a set of techniques to use with people with dementia. Others stress the phenomenological and humanistic perspective. Increasingly, it is also used interchangeably with a consumerist approach and personalisation.

The VIPS definition of person-centred care

The original VIPS definition (Brooker 2004) was a reaction to policy definitions in the UK at that time that were interpreting person-centred care simply as individualised care. This was in contrast to the ground-breaking work of the English academic Tom Kitwood in the 1990s, who had first used the term in the context of dementia care, which had emphasised the centrality of personhood and authentic communication. The VIPS definition was an attempt to spell out the different threads of person-centred care whilst maintaining the sophistication of Kitwood's original vision. It consisted of four essential elements (Brooker 2004).

- **Valuing** people with dementia and those who care for them: promoting their citizenship rights and entitlements regardless of age or cognitive impairment.

- Treating people as **individuals**: appreciating that all people with dementia have a unique history, identity, personality and physical, psychological, social and economic resources, and that these will affect their response to cognitive impairment.

- Looking at the world from the **perspective** of the person with dementia: recognising that each person's experience has its own psychological validity, that people with dementia act from this perspective and that empathy with this perspective has its own therapeutic potential.

- Recognising that all human life, including that of people with dementia, is grounded in relationships, and that people with dementia need an enriched **social environment** that both compensates for their impairment and fosters opportunities for personal growth.

These were simplified to:

V: A value base that asserts the absolute value of all human lives regardless of age or cognitive ability.

I: An individualised approach, recognising uniqueness.

P: Understanding the world from the perspective of the person identified as needing support.

S: Providing a social environment that supports psychological needs.

These four parts are called 'elements of person-centred care' in recognition of the fact that all these things can and do exist independently of each other. When they are brought together, however, they define a powerful approach to support personhood. Continuing the style that Tom Kitwood had for representing complex ideas in the form of equations, this can also be expressed as:

$$PCC \text{ (person-centred care)} = V + I + P + S$$

This equation does not give a pre-eminence of any element over another – they are all contributory. Of course, the acronym VIPs also stands for Very Important Persons, which is an easier way of defining the outcome of person-centred care for people with dementia.

The VIPS definition was used in the English NICE/SCIE (2007) guideline on dementia, which defined the principles of person-centred care as asserting:

- the human value of people with dementia, regardless of age or cognitive impairment, and those who care for them

- the individuality of people with dementia, with their unique personality and life experiences among the influences on their response to the dementia

- the importance of the perspective of the person with dementia

- the importance of relationships and interactions with others to the person with dementia, and their potential for promoting well-being.

(NICE/SCIE 2007, p.6)

The VIPS elements can be used as guiding principles for health and social care practitioners to reflect on their interactions with people with dementia and their families (Brooker 2012).

Reflective questions include:

- Does my behaviour and the manner in which I am communicating with this person show that I respect, value and honour them?

- Am I treating this person as a unique individual with a history and a wide range of strengths and needs?

- Am I making a serious attempt to see my actions from the perspective of the person I am trying to help? How might my actions be interpreted by this person?

- Do my behaviour and interactions help this person to feel socially confident and that they are not alone?

These principles apply in every situation where direct communication occurs. They apply when we are undertaking any health or social care intervention such as giving someone an injection, helping them to use the toilet, assisting them to complete an advance care plan or running a reminiscence group.

> It is not the task that is person-centred but the way in which that task is done.

The VIPS Framework for person-centred care services

This definition was used as the structure for the first edition of this book (Brooker 2007). This provided a set of concrete indicators against which care providers could benchmark their services. Pilot indicators were reviewed by around 50 care providers and service user organisations worldwide to arrive at a detailed description of what a person-centred care provider should have in place. This list of 25 indicators is grouped around the four elements of the definition set out above and has become known as the VIPS Framework.

These ideas in research and practice have continued to develop since this time. It has been taken up by many English-speaking care providers and the concepts have been translated into German, Japanese, Spanish, Norwegian and Portuguese. The VIPS Framework also underpins the Care Fit for VIPS website[1], a free web-based resource initially aimed at decreasing anti-psychotic use in care homes. Versions are also available for domiciliary care, day care and housing. It is also widely used by hospital and health staff.

We decided to write a second edition of this book because of the feedback we have had over the past ten years from service

---

1   www.carefitforvips.co.uk

providers worldwide. Time and time again people tell us that the VIPS Framework makes the delivery of person-centred care more manageable and deliverable, whilst recognising the complexity of the job in hand. This is not a quick fix or superficial solution, but neither is it mystical nor utopian. Person-centred care is not a single intervention but rather it is a set of guiding principles (VIPS) that suggests 25 ways that organisations can work to have an impact on the personhood of those receiving and delivering care.

Person-centred care requires sign-up to working in this way across the whole care provider organisation if it is to be sustained over any length of time. Particular elements require leadership at different levels.

- *Valuing elements of care* requires leadership from those responsible for leading the organisation at a senior level.

- *Individual care* requires leadership particularly from those responsible for setting care standards and procedures within the organisation.

- *Perspectives and social environment* requires leadership from those responsible for the day-to-day management and direct provision of care.

This framework enables care providers to break down the complexities of person-centred care into achievable steps. We have used it as part of our education courses for developing specialist practice in dementia care with over 2000 participants to date. Initially, course participants rate their service on each of the 25 indicators (using a simple scale of 'Excellent', 'Good', 'Okay' and 'Needs more work') in order to provide a profile of where they are doing well and what they need to improve upon. We then ask them to discuss this assessment with a variety of staff working at different levels within the organisation and with service users and carers where possible. Out of these discussions the managers and leaders learn a lot about the person-centredness of their organisation. As part of the education programme we then ask them to choose one or two areas that they have the ability and resources to work on to improve the quality of person-centred care.

The VIPS Framework has been adopted as a means of internally benchmarking the person-centredness of practice within a number of service settings, particularly within the care home sector. Baker (2014) describes utilising VIPS as an organising principle for an internal quality improvement programme (PEARL) in a large 'for-profit' care homes provider in the UK. In Norway, Rosvik and colleagues have developed the VIPS Practice Model as a means of improving quality of care for care homes residents (Røsvik *et al.* 2011, 2014). Rokstad *et al.* (2013) examined the impact of the VIPS Practice Model and Dementia Care Mapping when compared with usual dementia education sessions. Nursing home residents who were cared for by teams using the VIPS Practice Model showed significantly less depressive symptoms over time.

In the USA, Passalacqua and Harwood (2012) utilised the VIPS Framework to develop a series of workshops on improving communication skills of care workers in a large, for-profit, long-term, care facility. Using a pre-post evaluation, the course participants reported improved attitudes and skills as a result of the workshops.

The bedrock of VIPS: Tom Kitwood and person-centred care

One of the reasons why the VIPS Framework was developed was to build on the great work of the late Professor Tom Kitwood, an English academic who was a key figure in the theoretical development of person-centred approaches in dementia during the 1990s. Kitwood said that he first used the term 'person-centred' in relation to people with dementia to bring together ideas and ways of working with the lived experience of people with dementia that emphasised communication and relationships. The term was intended to be a direct reference to Rogerian psychotherapy (Rogers 1961) with its emphasis on authentic contact and communication.

Kitwood died at the age of 61 in 1998 just a year after the publication of his most well-known book *Dementia Reconsidered* (Kitwood 1997a), just as his theories were really beginning to gain traction in Europe, North America and Australia.

Kitwood's work was part of the groundswell of psychosocial approaches to dementia care that came into being during the 1980s and 1990s. Reality orientation (Holden and Woods 1988) was, in part, a response to offer reassurance to the person with dementia and a means of decreasing disorientation. Validation therapy (Feil 1993) and resolution therapy (Stokes and Goudie 1990) emphasised the importance of using the experience of the person with dementia as the starting point. Work on individualised care planning and social role valorisation, with its roots in the learning disabilities field, quickly caught on with those working in services for older people who were concerned with understanding the people they cared for at a deeper level and providing them with opportunities for leading a valued life.

The disability rights movement and the growing dissatisfaction with institutionalised care led to various codes of practice from the Kings Fund for England during the 1980s which emphasised the rights of people with dementia to live well. The work of Steven Sabat (Sabat 1994) was influential in shaping thinking about the impact of social environments on people with dementia. As far back as 1985, Joanne Rader and colleagues (Rader, Doan and Schwab 1985) used the term 'agenda behaviour' to highlight the goal seeking driving much of the behaviour of people with dementia. The Pioneer Network[2] in the USA has been working on changing the culture of long-term care for many years. The ideas of Bill Thomas and the Eden Alternative (Thomas 1996) gave the experience of older people in long-term care a centrality that was absent from approaches that had seen people as a set of problems to be managed.

The ideas that underpin person-centred approaches to care have been with us for a while. It is easy to forget how radical these ideas were when they were first described. Tom Kitwood provided a theoretical underpinning to the practice of person-centred dementia care. He published a continuous stream of articles in prominent journals during the 1980s and 1990s (Kitwood 1987a, 1987b, 1988, 1989, 1990a, 1990b, 1993a, 1993b, 1993c, 1995a, 1995b). The VIPS Framework sits squarely on the theoretical cornerstones developed by Kitwood: the importance of maintaining personhood; the Enriched Model of dementia; the recognition of the power of Malignant Social Psychology (MSP); striving to take the standpoint of the person living with dementia; and the description of New Culture care. In this opening chapter it is timely to review these.

---

2   http://pioneernetwork.net.

Personhood

Kitwood was also the first writer to use the term 'personhood' in relation to people living with dementia. He defined personhood as:

> A standing or status that is bestowed upon one human being, by others, in the context of relationship and social being. It implies recognition, respect and trust. (Kitwood 1997a, p.8)

The primary outcome of a person-centred approach is to maintain personhood in spite of the declining mental powers that dementia brings. There is an assumption in person-centred care that people living with dementia have the capacity to experience relative well-being and ill-being throughout the course of their experience of dementia. A simplistic biological model would interpret the expression of ill-being as a random occurrence or as a sign of brain pathology. In person-centred care, the assumption is made that behaviour has meaning. According to Kitwood, high levels of challenging behaviour, distress or apathy occur more commonly in care settings that are not supportive of personhood. In care environments that are supportive of personhood, we expect to see a greater preponderance of well-being and social confidence.

Person-centred care aims to maintain and nurture personhood. Personhood is what makes us essentially human. It is what human beings recognise in each other and it engenders feelings of trust, security and well-being between people at whatever age or ability level. There is a high level of risk that people living with dementia are treated as if they are 'non-persons'. The risk of this is greater when the level of impairment is more advanced. The historical narrative that 'dementia is the death that leaves the body behind' has been vigorously challenged over the past 20 years but is still prevalent in many societies and communities. It may sometimes be difficult to see the personhood in others who have advanced dementia but the assumption is made that it is always there to be found.

This theme runs through this book but it is picked up particularly in Chapters 3 and 4 when we consider how people living with dementia are valued by society generally, and how care providers need to make the valuing of the quality of life into explicit business if they are serious about providing person-centred care.

The Enriched Model of dementia

Tom Kitwood described the Enriched Model of dementia. This challenged the prevailing assumption in the 1980s that dementia could be understood simply by the degree of loss of brain cortex, what Kitwood called 'the standard paradigm'. The Enriched Model recognised the multiplicity of factors that affect a person's experience of dementia, including neurological impairment, physical health, the individual's biography and personality, and the social environment in which they live. At the time when Kitwood first wrote about the Enriched Model, it was thought that little could be done to arrest neurological impairment. The Enriched Model provided the opportunity to maximise well-being by focusing on the other dimensions that affect a person's quality of life. The person-centred approach sees dementia as a condition that needs to be understood from a biological, a psychological and a sociological (bio-psycho-social) perspective, and to recognise that all these perspectives interact to determine the person's experience of the condition. This theme of the uniqueness of experience is discussed in Chapter 4 when we look at the necessity of providing individualised care for those receiving services if their needs are to be supported in a way that is person-centred.

Malignant Social Psychology (MSP)

Personhood is undermined when individual needs and rights are not considered, when powerful negative emotions are ignored or invalidated and when increasing isolation from human relationships occurs. Kitwood described the various common ways that he had observed personhood being undermined in care settings, coining the phrase 'Malignant Social Psychology' (MSP) as an umbrella term. MSP includes episodes where people are intimidated, outpaced, not responded to, infantilised, labelled, disparaged, blamed, manipulated, invalidated, disempowered, overpowered, disrupted, objectified, stigmatised, ignored, banished and mocked. Very few people would wish to deliberately subject other people to MSP. Despite this, in the care of people living with dementia around the world, it occurs with surprising regularity. The MSP list is a depressingly familiar one to people working in care. Many care practitioners have a heart-sink feeling when they first read this list.

Kitwood was at pains to say that episodes of MSP are very rarely done with any malicious intent. Rather, episodes of MSP become interwoven into the care culture. When these ways of behaving are seen repeatedly, they become unquestioned and normalised and part of the organisational culture. This way of responding to people with dementia gets learnt in the same way that new staff learn to fold sheets. If you are a new staff member on a hospital ward, you learn how to communicate with patients by following the example set by other staff with whom you work. If their communication style with patients is one that is characterised by infantilisation and outpacing, then you will follow their lead. The malignancy in MSP is that it eats away at the personhood of those being cared for, and also that it spreads from one member of staff to another very quickly.

Frequent episodes of MSP undermine personhood, decrease well-being and increase ill-being. Kitwood postulated that the increasing isolation that resulted from MSP could in itself lead to a loss of function. At its worst, it leads to a radical depersonalisation of people living with dementia, and reconfirms to wider society its belief that those living with the condition are less in need of love and support.

The root of MSP lies within our societal values. People with dementia are not valued in societies where youth and intellectual prowess receive the highest accolades. In care settings, this lack of value manifests itself as MSP. The impact of MSP is picked up in Chapter 6 when we consider the importance of promoting a positive social environment in care services for people living with dementia.

The standpoint of the person with dementia

One of Kitwood's main concerns was to try to understand the experience of care from the standpoint of the person living with dementia. Much of Kitwood's own understanding of dementia came from spending time talking to people experiencing dementia or time observing life in care homes and day centres. His early versions of Dementia Care Mapping (DCM) were an attempt to evaluate care from the perspective of the person living with dementia (Kitwood and Bredin 1992a). Later versions emphasised the developmental nature of these evaluations as a driver for the development of person-centred care. Kitwood described DCM as 'a serious attempt to take the standpoint of the person with dementia, using a combination of empathy and observational skill' (1997a, p.4). The centrality of engaging directly with the experience of people living with dementia began to find prominence in the 1990s. The theme is picked up in Chapter 5 when we consider the importance of ensuring that the perspective of the person living with dementia is taken as the starting point in providing person-centred care.

New Culture of care

Kitwood also described the Old Culture–New Culture shift in relation to dementia care services (Kitwood and Benson 1995). Many points that he discussed as being part of the New Culture have also become included in person-centred care. New Culture care encompasses the following points:

- Dementia care work is seen as a creative and dynamic option rather than unskilled work that no one wants.

- Dementia is seen as a disability to be lived with, rather than a disease process to be managed.

- People with dementia and those who care for them on a day-to-day basis have an expertise of their own to report upon that is as important as brain science.

- All people are equal regardless of cognitive ability.

- The task of care is the maintenance of personhood and that the uniqueness and individuality of all is recognised regardless of diagnosis.

- Problem behaviours are seen primarily as attempts at communication.

- Care work is recognised as emotional work, and it is clear that staff caring for people with dementia need to have their own personhood respected if they are to do a good job.

Culture of care is key

Over recent years there has been much more attention paid to the impact of the culture of care on service quality in hospitals and care homes. Staff burnout has been shown to be associated with less willingness to help residents, low optimism and negative emotional responses to their behaviour (Todd and Watts 2005). High levels of staff turnover, staff shortages and poorly trained staff exacerbated feelings of depression in care home residents (Choi, Ransom and Wyllie 2008). There is evidence to suggest that staff groups who have received training and ongoing support in delivering person-centred care show positive outcomes (CSCI 2008; Chenoweth et al. 2009; Deudon et al. 2009; Fossey et al. 2006) and that beliefs about the personhood of people with dementia influence staff behaviour (Hunter et al. 2013). Studies have also reported that person-centred interventions lead to decreased job stress and strain as well as increased personal and professional satisfaction (McKeown et al. 2010; Jeon et al. 2012). Understanding the culture of care and what aspects impact on the provision of person-centredness show the interconnectedness of relationships between those in receipt of care, those who work in care and those who manage and direct care (Kirkley et al. 2011).

In this second edition we will be drawing heavily on a large-scale research programme (the CHOICE project (Care Home Organisations Implementing Cultures of Excellence) Killett et al. 2014) that unpicked the key positive features of care cultures that supported personhood in people with advanced dementia and complex needs in care homes. We were both privileged to work on this programme and we learnt a lot from care teams and people living with dementia about what really helps to maintain personhood. The features that this study clarified are described in depth in Chapter 2.

Dementia is a global issue

Since the 2007 first edition there has been a sea change in the recognition of the needs of people living with dementia in a way that we would not have thought possible back then. An increasing number of countries now have National Dementia Strategies. There is evidence that these national strategies really do have an impact on front-line care (Edvardsson, Sandman and Borell 2014). The world at last appears to be waking up to the fact that the numbers of people living with dementia makes it a significant public health issue. The number of people estimated to be living with dementia worldwide in 2013 was 44.35 million. This is predicted to rise to 75.62 million in 2030 and 135.46 million in 2050 (Alzheimer's Disease International 2010). Alzheimer's Disease International (2010) estimates that by 2050, 71 per cent of people living with dementia worldwide will live in low- and middle-income countries.

At a global level, the first Ministerial Conference on Global Action Against Dementia was held by the World Health Organization in 2015 where 80 countries signed a call to action to improve the quality of life for people living with dementia. Some global action focuses on trying to find a cure for dementia and promoting lifestyles to reduce the numbers getting dementia. However, there is much concern that the increasing numbers of people living with dementia need care and support that is person-centred, and recommendations about developing services that support people from pre-diagnosis through to end-of-life are available (OECD 2015). This includes dementia-friendly communities, timely diagnosis, post diagnostic support programmes, end-of-life care and psycho-social and public health interventions.

There is much to celebrate in that the needs of people whose lives are affected by dementia are now achieving recognition. This has been accelerated by the significant numbers of people living with dementia advocating on their own behalf. The rights to be aware of diagnosis and treatment options are at the forefront of national and international policy. The increasing recognition that the voices of those living with dementia need to be heard directly in shaping and developing services has become an accepted way of working, if not always easy to achieve in practice. More and more direct accounts of what it is like to live with dementia are now accessible through social media, books, TV and films.

One of the first accounts came from the Australian writer, Christine Bryden, in her book *Dancing with Dementia* (2005), who we featured in the first edition of this book. Christine was formerly a top civil servant who was diagnosed with dementia at the age of 46. Ten years later, Christine described her journey with dementia as a dance, whereby both she and her husband, Paul, have had to change their steps along the way to form the pattern of the dance. Twenty years on from her original diagnosis, Christine Bryden is still writing and advocating on behalf of people living with dementia worldwide but now she is joined by many others. Her insights from ten years ago remain as pertinent as ever and we have retained many of her original quotes from *Dancing with Dementia* throughout this book to illustrate key points about person-centred care.

> Each person with dementia is travelling a journey deep into the core of their spirit, away from the complex cognitive outer layer that once defined them, through the jumble and tangle of emotions created through their life experiences, into the centre of their being, into what truly gives them meaning in life. Many of us seek earnestly for this sense of the present time, the sense of 'now', of how to live each moment and treasure it as if it were the only experience to look at and to wonder at. But this is the experience of dementia, life in the present without a past or future. (Bryden 2005, p.11)

Person-centred care and the ideas that influence it continue to grow. In many respects, these ideas no longer seem radical. The challenge remains, however, of how we get these ideas into everyday practice. Whilst the amount of policy initiatives, policy guidelines and research evidence supporting person-centred approaches is growing, the gap between the rhetoric and the reality remains wide in many cases. No single country has found a solution for how we manage this on a large scale, although many have islands of good practice. This is a global challenge and demands a global response in the same way as finding a cure for dementia.

The person-centred care provider

Person-centred care is a term that has become common parlance in dementia care. The ideas behind it no longer seem radical but its practice is often ill defined and difficult to evidence. Although the many contexts and interventions that are involved in skilled care will vary worldwide we believe that the universal challenge that faces people living with dementia is that their personhood is undermined by poor quality care and support. By ensuring that people can preserve their personhood and have the opportunity to remain in relationship with their environment, they can maintain independence, autonomy, personal growth, joy, pleasure, meaningful activity, life satisfaction, fulfilment and a sense of well-being.

In this opening chapter, we have reviewed the origins of person-centred care as defined by Tom Kitwood and others who have followed in his wake. In this new edition we have also included a new chapter that focuses on the issue of care culture. The VIPS definition of person-centred care is a four-part composite. The basis for this is reviewed in the remaining chapters of Part 1. In Part 2 we describe the VIPS Framework. The Framework consists of six key indicators for each of the VIPS elements. This can be used for care providers of different kinds to evidence their practice. VIPS is designed to help care providers think through the issues in the provision of person-centred care in a systematic way. Providing good-quality person-centred care is not an easy undertaking. It becomes more straightforward, however, if we can articulate and clearly describe what it is we are doing as dementia-care providers to ensure that our services are person-centred.

2

Organisational Culture and Person-centred Dementia Care

Care culture is something that people recognise through its impact rather than by its definition. Its impact is what people sense when they walk through the door of a care home, hospital ward or GP surgery or when an assessment is carried out by a domiciliary care manager or social worker. The impact of culture is often what people are attempting to grasp when they 'can't put a finger on' what feels right or wrong about a place or situation. Whilst good care culture may be hard to define, people generally know it when they see it. In fact, more accurately, people know it when they *don't* see it.

In the distressing and ever more common exposés of poor care, whether in care homes, hospitals or people's own homes, the 'culture' pervading an organisation or workforce is often cited as both cause and solution. However, this is spoken of as a taken-for-granted idea, one that everyone understands, without ever focusing on the details of day-to-day processes and underlying dynamics that create, reinforce or discourage the actions (or inactions) that result in poor care. Robert Francis QC, the chair of the public inquiry into the failures of Mid Staffordshire NHS Foundation Trust went so far as to suggest that blaming 'culture' is the response used 'when no one can think of anything else' (Francis 2011). It seems that while people are increasingly certain of its importance, they still struggle to put their finger on what 'it' actually entails.

Within the care sector, leaders and managers are very often surprised at what does (or does not) emerge as a result of their efforts to change care practice. This is because they may not have considered the impact that care culture may have on what can (or cannot) change on the ground. If leaders and managers truly wish to achieve a person-centred approach for people living with dementia then they need to be able to recognise the features and impact of culture on actions and behaviours in care delivery. They need to find ways to influence it positively. Without such understanding there is a risk that efforts to improve care will fail to have maximum impact or create only temporary enthusiasm rather than long-term change.

What is culture?

One look at the *Oxford English Dictionary*'s definition of the word 'culture' shows it has many overlapping meanings. It is used in diverse contexts and situations and is familiar to gardeners, business leaders and history professors alike. However, there is a common thread through all those definitions: culture is the all-pervasive substance in which we grow. It is where we have our roots and from where we absorb our nourishment. Whether it is the culture of our workplace, community, organisation or society, we take up and use what is available to us from our cultural soil, good or bad. Crucially, we cannot help but soak it up. We do it inevitably, often unconsciously, and we cannot separate ourselves from that soil. What is in the soil affects how well we can grow, regardless of how much pruning and attention we receive from outside. Therefore, if we wish to grow and if we want to help people to live well with dementia, we need to pay attention to what we are all absorbing from our cultural soil.

Services for people living with dementia exist within the context of society. People living with dementia face societal challenges because of the stigma and prejudice towards people who are dependent through age and poor health. This stigma and prejudice impact on people living with dementia, their families and those who provide care and services. It impacts on how society values and prioritises (or fails to prioritise) care work. We will return to this in Chapter 4 when we consider the first important element of the VIPS Framework, 'Valuing'.

It is beyond the scope of most of us to change the world. However, we can change the organisational culture in which we work if we take the time to understand it and the influence it has on person-centred care.

Organisational culture

Research into 'organisational culture', its interaction and impact on success, leadership and management has been an ever-expanding field of study since the 1970s. However, it is notable that it has taken a long time for this research and the insights it offers to be considered in relation to health and social care settings. Maybe this is based on the belief that the good-heartedness of those working in the care field is enough to ensure the culture is a good one; that this provides an adequate soil that caring professionals and those who come into contact with them need. When neglectful or abusive practice occurs, the first reaction is often to focus on the individual who is seen as responsible at the front line. The cries of 'rotten apples' and assertions that, 'Well, *I* would never do that,' abound in response to the undercover documentary or government inquiry. However, our experience of years of working in care settings suggests that this is wishful thinking at best and turning a blind eye at worst. The healthiest and most fruitful of plants will wither if placed in poor soil.

Perhaps our reluctance to transfer learning about organisational culture into the field of care also comes from a reluctance to equate the world of 'care' with the world of 'business'. We would suggest that this reluctance is misplaced, and not simply because the provision of care is increasingly carried out as a business. It is important to recognise that there are lessons to be learnt from business research. If the owner of a computer software business sees fit to explore how the dynamics and processes of their organisation affects their output, then we should certainly want to explore how such organisational dynamics and processes affect the outcomes of care. Poor organisational culture in a computer software company results only in malfunctioning software and a failing business. Poor organisational culture in care results in profound unhappiness, neglect and ill-being for the most vulnerable and, ultimately, a failing society.

Phillip Zimbardo, a social psychologist famous for research into why and how (and how easily) good people can do bad things has highlighted that the factors responsible are not primarily about individual 'bad apples' but, more crucially, are embedded in organisational, structural and societal influences; 'bad barrels' and 'bad barrel-makers' (Zimbardo 2007). Kitwood recognised this in his call to transform from the 'Old Culture' to a 'New Culture' of care. In describing the behaviours observed in care settings that detracted from well-being of people living with dementia he emphasised that, in the majority of instances, these were not done deliberately or maliciously but were rather habitual actions, passed from one worker to another and normalised in the day-to-day conduct of caring work (Kitwood 1997a). In this, he began to describe the process and influence of organisational culture on the care outcomes that any workplace, service or organisation produces. He was highlighting the need to think about these processes and their influence, rather than focus attention solely on describing 'good outcomes' and instructing individuals. Crucially, he recognised that there is a need to work actively towards such positive cultures, rather than merely hoping that they would emerge from people's good will and knowledge.

Many descriptions of organisational culture exist, focusing on different aspects and their influence in a variety of different fields. What emerges from these descriptions and attempts to apply them in practice is an understanding that organisational culture is more than a single issue, such as the aims or purpose of an organisation, the management style used or the skills and motivations of individual workers. It is, instead, a product of all of these factors and more, interacting on a day-to-day basis, influencing the decision-making and problem-solving of daily work and fortifying or undermining each other at every turn.

In seeking to describe the complexity of organisational culture, Schein (1990) explained it as the assumptions shared by members of an organisation, used in their daily practice, and reinforced through providing successful solutions to problems faced in the course of work. Crucially, these assumptions are passed on to new members of the organisation as the 'right' way to view and carry out their work, thereby perpetuating and further embedding such assumptions. This may, initially, seem to be a complex explanation, but anyone who has worked, lived or visited care services will have experienced the 'it's the way we do things here' speech as part of their induction, in discussion with colleagues or as a response to questioning an approach that seems inexplicable to a newcomer or outsider. Many of us have experienced the uncomfortable moment when we realise we have transformed unintentionally from the questioning newcomer into the old timer who tells others that 'this is the way we do it here'. This is organisational culture in action.

It is this unintentional transformation that signals why understanding and seeking to influence the various aspects of organisational culture matter so much. Habits become habits because they are useful to us; they help us to solve problems and respond to changes easily and successfully. Old habits are hard to break precisely because people do not recognise them as habits. They are carried out unthinkingly and when they are questioned it can seem impossible and feel threatening to think of an alternative: after all, if this isn't the best way to do it, why have I been doing it this way all along?

To create and sustain change towards truly person-centred care, it is important to harness everything that has the potential to influence the way the day-to-day work of person-centred care is carried out. This means thinking about the different forces that act on the ground to encourage, permit or discourage person-centred solutions being the response to the day-to-day challenges and changes inherent to caring well for a person with dementia. These forces come from the physical and social environment in which care is carried out, the values that are embedded in the way people think and feel about their work and the behaviour that is acceptable, allowable or encouraged through the patterns and rewards of work in an organisation. All of these can help to reinforce or contradict what we want to achieve by influencing those assumptions and habits that become embedded in day-to-day practice.

What happens when we do not consider organisational culture? An example from practice

The view from the Board of Trustees

At The Brilliant Care Company we have recently invested heavily in recruiting and training our staff and refining our care plans with the intention of achieving more person-centred care. This has taken huge amounts of money, time and effort from senior staff in the organisation. However, this has not had the impact we had hoped for. We are demotivated and some of us blame the front-line staff and managers for the failure. After all, we did so much to try and help them!

The view from the front line

As a care worker in one of the care homes run by The Brilliant Care Company there are many factors that influence the way I work. Chief among these are what is seen as 'success' on a daily basis, alongside what is encouraged and discouraged by others who work in or visit the home. If these are not changed then the efforts of the company at a higher level will amount to nothing. My personal wish may be to promote happiness and well-being for my residents, and my training may tell me this too, but if I am congratulated for getting lunch completed on time, if the physical environment means I have to keep people in a certain room even if they want to move or if I am criticised by the visiting doctor for allowing someone to lie in, then it will not be long before I develop assumptions and habits that counter truly person-centred care. It is expecting too much of anyone to require that I regularly experience, let alone resist, such contradictory pressures. To me, it feels as if The Brilliant Care Company do not understand what it is like to do my job, and they do not appreciate me. After all, if they did, they would try to help me, not make things harder!

If we wish to improve the care and support for people living with dementia that is provided by health and social care organisations such as care homes, hospitals, GP surgeries, and home-care services then we must address all the things that influence 'the way we do things here' for that individual service and organisation. That requires openness, honesty and critical reflection on what we do, the way we do it and why that may be the case. It demands more than simply stating where we wish to be or telling front-line staff or regulators what it should look like. We have to explore what *is*, listen to those on the front line (both receiving care and delivering it) about *why* it is and then work together to ensure that everything an organisation does reinforces the right assumptions and habits and makes the wrong ones untenable in practice. We have to reflect on our role in all of it, whether we are a front-line worker, a manager, an inspector, a visitor, a government minister, a business owner or a university professor.

Getting to a person-centred care culture in an organisation takes courage and effort and sustaining it requires even more. It requires individuals and groups to challenge constantly what is 'normal' and accepted in an organisation and to be willing to risk trying out new ways of working. The VIPS Framework as outlined in this book is designed to help, encourage and give you confidence with this. The next section identifies the particular elements of organisational culture that are important for person-centred care to flourish.

New Culture of care revisited

In Chapter 1 we described Kitwood's vision of the New Culture of dementia care and how important he saw this as a means of establishing person-centred care. We want to build on this idea by adding to it the findings of a recent research project in which we were involved. The CHOICE project (Care Home Organisations Implementing Cultures of Excellence) emerged from a programme of research exploring the features, causes and preventative factors related to the institutional abuse of older adults, including those with dementia (Lupton and Croft-White 2013). The particular focus of the CHOICE project was to establish the factors that created positive cultures, recognising that this was an area that we knew little about (Killett *et al.* 2014). It is vitally important that we can describe what a positive care culture is and how it is achieved, as well as identify poor and abusive care when it occurs. If we do not highlight both ends of this spectrum there is a danger that we focus only on punitive measures to prevent the bad and assume that anything that is 'not bad' is automatically good.

There is a long way between 'satisfactory' and 'outstanding'. Mediocre is not enough when we are talking about people in need of continued, skilled support to counteract the impact of cognitive decline. Only excellence will do. This is care fit for VIPS: Very Important Persons. Excellence supports Personhood. Mediocrity just about keeps people alive.

We worked on CHOICE with colleagues from three other UK universities. Our researchers spent a prolonged period of time (over three months) in 11 different care homes across England, Wales and Scotland. The homes were very mixed in terms of size, location, owning organisation and registration. We undertook an in-depth case study in each home that involved observing the care experience and interviewing residents, staff, managers and visitors. In effect, we were trying to get underneath the skin of the home in order to understand the deeper organisational culture.

Often when researchers or regulators try to understand a care home they begin by interviewing the managers or owners. We took a rather different approach in our research. The first task in the research was to use an observation tool (*PIECE-dem*, Brooker *et al.* 2013) to uncover the experiences of the residents with advanced dementia and complex needs. This meant that the first introduction to care in the home was through the eyes of those people who had very limited communication or sensory or physical difficulties in addition to their dementia. Subsequent observations and interviews tried to understand the culture in the care home that influenced the experiences of the most vulnerable and dependent in the home.

Using a comparative case study design (Eisenhardt and Graebner 2007), guided by the structures described by Schein (1990), the research team identified seven key features of positive care cultures that had a significant bearing on how people experienced care. These features are all connected to each other and are described in the rest of this chapter. Whilst the results and examples from CHOICE that we share in this book are care home based, our experience suggests that the features of care culture that impact on people living with dementia and complex needs may also be important to consider in hospitals, home care and primary care. We have also used examples from a broader range of service provision to illustrate these features.

CHOICE was a serious research endeavour and as such the language used to describe the findings may seem overly complex to those not used to reading research papers. What these features illustrate, however, is far from obscure. The findings resonate with all of us who have known good care. Put simply the findings are thus:

> We all **work together** to deliver the best care. **We all matter** to each other. We **empower and support front-line staff** to empower and support people living with dementia. Our leadership **protects front-line service delivery** as paramount. On a day-to-day basis this means that every day is different and staff **constantly look to make things better** for the people they care for. We help people to **enjoy places where they spend time** and to be **active in a way that fulfils them every day**.

We illustrate this with a picture in Figure 2.1.

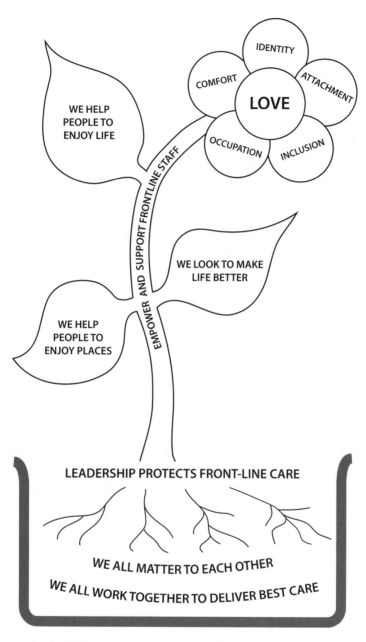

Figure 2.1 The fulfilment of psychological needs (Kitwood 1997a) depends on a positive care culture – A pictorial representation of how the elements of a positive care culture can support the emotional and psychological well-being of people living with dementia in a care setting

Feature 1: A practical, shared purpose in providing person-centred care

We all work together to deliver the best care.

As noted elsewhere in this book, talk of person-centred care abounds. There is scarcely a care home, hospital or government guideline nowadays that does not espouse the intention of 'person-centred' care. However, intentions are not sufficient by themselves. In fact, good intentions can often mask uncertainty and contradiction by providing a glossy veneer that distracts attention away from real-life experiences on the ground. A shared purpose in providing person-centred care goes far beyond talk and is exhibited by anyone and everyone involved in the organisation in two key ways.

First, a shared purpose means that there is a consistency in understanding between all involved in the organisation (from executive management to visitors and front-line staff) as to what 'good care' should look and feel like on the ground. In particular, this understanding relates to practical, everyday experiences of people receiving care, rather than relying on an overarching definition or intention. Without this practical basis, individuals and groups within an organisation can develop different and sometimes contradictory aims, each in the belief that they have the 'right' or 'best' interpretation. The reason this shared and practical explanation of purpose is so important for a positive organisational culture is not that it magically makes person-centred care easy to achieve. Instead, it is that it provides a shared framework that can be used to consider, resolve and learn from the challenges, problems and opportunities presented by the ever-changing day-to-day practice when working with people.

A practical example of shared purpose: A good day for Bob

Imagine Bob's care home. It strives to provide person-centred care, but this has been translated for everyone in contact with the care home into what it practically means for Bob in his daily life. A good day for Bob is understood as (amongst many other things) a chance to watch, talk or play football. When this is the shared definition of person-centred care that everyone who influences the life of the home works towards it becomes much easier to facilitate and to reflect on success (or lack of success) in achieving it. If Bob did not chat about football yesterday, why did he not? What needs to change tomorrow to make sure he can if he wants to? If he had a fabulous time watching the match, what made that happen and how can we do it again? It provides a clear framework against which daily practice and organisational decisions can be judged: did they help or hinder Bob (and each of his neighbours) to have a good day? How do we know? If not, why not, and what has to change?

Without such a practical explanation, challenges and difficulties are harder to resolve and lessons harder to learn, because it is harder to pinpoint the exact nature of the problem. If we do not know specifically what we are aiming for, how can we know if and why we missed the target? Did Bob miss the football match because the staff could not be bothered or because they could not be in two places at once? Was it because the kitchen routine meant Bob (and his support staff) had to make a choice between watching the match and eating dinner? Was it because activities in this home take place according to a predetermined schedule and the match is not amongst them? Was it because the environment means Bob cannot watch TV without irritating his football-hating neighbour? A shared framework of 'Bob's good day involves football' helps us to answer these questions. A lack of a shared framework means we could struggle to work out what did or did not work. Moreover, without such a practical and shared understanding there is a real risk that the *appearance* of a good day (a tidy room, an activities schedule, all physical care being provided, dinner being served on time) could be confused for the *experience* of a good day. We might never find out whether Bob had a good day or not.

The second way an organisation with a positive culture enables this shared and practical view of person-centred care is through the interactions that take place between and with staff in that organisation. If a manager knows what constitutes a good day for the front-line workers, where their skills and struggles lie, then the manager can encourage and enable them to use and develop those skills and support them when they have a bad day. This requires the manager to listen to, get to know and value the staff. It requires *their* manager to listen to, get to know and value them. Mirroring the practical experience of person-centred care in day-to-day interactions throughout an organisation is crucial to helping its implementation and sustenance in care-giving interactions. If a member of staff feels unheard, devalued and unsupported, how can we expect them to listen closely, value deeply and support joyfully the needs of people living with dementia? Being truly present and attentive to anyone, particularly someone living with the challenges dementia can bring, is an emotionally, physically and intellectually demanding task. Therefore the interactions and structure of the organisation around us must recognise, empathise with and actively support staff in achieving it.

Feature 2: Connectedness and community between all involved in the organisation

> We all matter to each other.

This feature is about the extent to which everyone involved in the organisation feels part of things within the organisation and is linked to the external community. Whether you are an employee, volunteer, visitor, neighbour or person living with dementia, a positive care culture encourages your participation in the organisation and values the contributions you can make to it, big or small. It is about efforts to encourage individual caring connections and a positive atmosphere between people involved with the organisation, whether as worker, visitor or person receiving care and support.

Connectedness is important in creating a positive care culture for the people receiving care for a number of reasons. If a sense of connectedness exists between and across different 'functions' within the organisation, it helps the organisation develop and sustain that shared purpose described above in a constant and ongoing way. Without it, organisational decision-making, day-to-day practice and people's experiences are disconnected from each other, or only connected through infrequent formalised routes such as complaints procedures, supervision meetings or consultation events. Connectedness ensures investment in that organisation and its people and a sense of responsibility and ownership of what goes on within it. This results in an active involvement and contribution to that organisation and a constructive engagement when problems or difficulties arise. Without connectedness, a person cannot see or find a way to contribute their skills and abilities, has no such sense of investment and is more likely to engage only when and if it is necessary to achieve their own needs without consideration of the whole community.

A practical example of connectedness: Care for Mrs Komar at home

Imagine that Mrs Komar uses a care agency to provide her with personal care on a daily basis. The owner, manager and staff know about the importance of everyone involved with the agency feeling connected and having a sense of how they can participate to the best of their abilities. This means that, as well as making sure their assessments and care arrangements meet the (person-centred) needs of Mrs Komar, they also seek out and try to understand the experiences of Mrs Komar's daughter as her informal carer. They invite informal carers to an open evening and share information about additional support there is in the local area. At the event, informal carers meet others in similar situations and get to meet some of the care workers. Mrs Komar's care worker and daughter share how much they love it when they can encourage Mrs Komar to pick up her knitting needles, and this starts a discussion about how loneliness and boredom can be a real challenge for someone with dementia. From this comes the idea to try to meet for a 'knit and natter' coffee morning and one of the care workers suggests a café in town that is accessible and friendly. When it is successful, plans turn to how they could find a way to have some extra 'time off' for themselves and enjoyable company for their family member. When they need some professional support, they turn to the care agency first and foremost, as they know the staff team has the enthusiasm and skills to make it work.

Whilst this sort of scenario might feel as if it's pie in the sky, it is what can emerge from connected organisations, where every opportunity is taken to encourage interaction, understanding and participation for people, regardless of their particular 'role'. In a disconnected home-care agency Mrs Komar's daughter feels that her only role is to check that the care worker has completed the visit properly. The care worker sees her responsibility only in relation to Mrs Komar and feels untrusted and underappreciated by Mrs Komar's daughter. The manager then has to take responsibility for fielding Mrs Komar's daughter's calls and addressing any problems with the care worker. It is easy to see how, in this alternate disconnected culture, problems fester and frustrations rise rather than difficulties being identified and problems being solved. Most importantly, Mrs Komar herself may well get lost even though everyone has her care in mind. In this scenario, her care may be appropriate and acceptable, but she will never get to have a weekly cuppa at a coffee shop in the company of new friends.

Feature 3: Staff are empowered to take responsibility for the well-being of people receiving care and are supported to do so through active management processes

We empower and support front-line staff.

This feature is about is the way in which front-line staff approach the day-to-day work with people they support and, significantly, the ways in which this is encouraged and enabled by the approach and practices of management and leaders within a particular workplace. Front-line workers in positive care cultures are enabled to go about their work in two interconnected ways. First, they are responsible in what they do: they have care and concern for the people they are supporting, an understanding of their duty and accountability for their work. Second, they are autonomous within their work: they are able to take decisions and carry out actions for the benefit of a person they are supporting because they have the necessary skills, support and freedom to act within the remit of their particular role. Crucially, it is both of these *together* that matters rather than one or the other.

It is not sufficient to recruit and train for 'responsible' staff without thinking about how to empower them. If staff in a workplace are only responsible, they may care deeply but not be able to do what they know is important for the people they support because the organisation, often unintentionally, gets in the way. They can see what someone needs, but have no power to make it happen. Decisions are made elsewhere, without real consultation and the staff's responsibility is to enact those decisions, regardless of how it impacts on people receiving care. Staff in these situations will burn out, become frustrated or have to downgrade their expectations about what can be achieved on behalf of the people they support. On the other hand, autonomous staff who are not responsible have great freedom to act and influence decisions and actions on a day-to-day basis, but it will not necessarily be used to benefit people receiving support because the underlying sense of care, concern or understanding of duty is absent. Staff in these situations may do what is best for themselves or enact poor understanding of what is good for the people they support.

This is where management and leadership practices are crucial in enabling staff to be both responsible and autonomous in their work. Without such practices (and constant reflection on their impact) then the culture in a particular workplace will inadvertently create a situation in which staff cannot be both or are encouraged to be one but not the other. This will and does result in less than positive experiences for people receiving care and support. The practices, approach and behaviours that matter in encouraging both responsibility and autonomy from staff are listed below.

Managers and leaders are:

- supportive of staff needs, both practical and emotional

- responsive and encouraging of staff input and requests

- present in the setting where and when the care and support takes place

- seen to lead by example in their interactions with staff, visitors and people receiving support

- able to define clearly the boundaries of different roles in the setting

- strong and united when making decisions or taking action.

This may seem as if it is an overwhelming list for those managers among you! However, it is important to remember that 'management and leadership' are not about one single role in an organisation. They are about a variety of people and roles, which will differ depending on the type and purpose of an organisation and the skills of those involved. A manager is not able to be everywhere at once but a team of people in different positions, different roles and with different skills can be. We mention both 'management and leadership' here to highlight that whilst some roles may be specified within an organisation, others may be more informal, but nonetheless influential through their contact and role-modelling to others. Leadership and management are different things, and as such, creating the right organisational culture to encourage and enable the right attitudes and behaviours of staff does not, and should not, fall on the shoulders of only one person.

A practical example of empowered and enabled staff: Day opportunities for Mr Stephens

Mr Stephens attends a day centre. The staff here are employed, encouraged and rewarded for their passion, care and concern for people living with dementia (they are responsible). They are also skilled and supported to make decisions and act in the situations that arise in the course of their work (they are autonomous). Mr Stephens is a regular attendee who benefits from the chance it gives his partner to continue to work. However, on some days he can become quite restless and loud and try to leave the centre.

Mike, a support worker, knows that there could be lots of reasons for this and so begins to try and find out why. He offers to go for a walk with Mr Stephens as soon as he goes to the door. His team leader tells him to call if he has any problems and then steps in to help the other staff at lunchtime when Mike would have helped with serving food. The cook notices that Mr Stephens is not there for lunch and so puts a suitable meal to one side for him.

When Mr Stephens and Mike return, the team leader thanks Mike and tells him to take a break while she gets Mr Stephens' lunch. The day-centre manager chats with Mike at the end of the shift to see what happened. Mike tells her that Mr Stephens was more relaxed outside but hard to encourage back inside, as he kept worrying about all the flowerbeds along the road. He wonders if Mr Stephens might be bored, as many of the other day-centre attendees are women.

They decide that a discussion with Mr Stephens' partner might be helpful and the manager agrees to do it the next day. She reports back to Mike and the team leader that Mr Stephens used to spend a lot of time at his allotment. The team leader suggests that Mike thinks about some ways that Mr Stephens could get involved with gardening, reminding him that another worker has an allotment.

Within a few weeks, Mike has organised getting some second-hand plant tubs and negotiated some free plants and seeds from a local garden centre in exchange for an advert on the centre's front door. Every day Mr Stephen's arrives with his gardening gloves and a trowel. The chef provides soup in a flask for lunch, which Mr Stephens eats by the back door when he takes a break from his day's work. The manager and team leader are planning an event to raise some funds to get a proper garden set up at the centre.

This example shows how important both a sense of responsibility and freedom to act on that responsibility are for all of the staff working at the centre, regardless of their role.

Without responsibility, no one will notice Mr Stephens' distress or undertake to solve some of the difficulties it might cause him (missing lunch, trying to leave the centre or disturbing others). Without autonomy, individual workers may have a strong desire to help but they cannot do so because they are not allowed to. They are restricted from leaving the centre because of concerns about risk or staffing levels, and they are not asked for their opinion about what will work or encouraged to implement those ideas. They are criticised when they do something differently to see if it will work, or they are prohibited because they have to wait for advice and permission or receive contradictory information from different sources. In both scenarios, Mr Stephens' well-being will suffer and the staff's work could become stressful, frustrating and dissatisfying as a result.

Feature 4: Management mediates the impact of
external factors on front-line care delivery

Our leadership protects front-line care delivery.

This feature highlights the significance of external factors and how they are managed by and within an organisation. External factors are anything from outside of the organisation or specific workplace that can have an impact on the day-to-day practice of staff and thus the support of people living with dementia. These could include things such as:

- regulatory/statutory requirements and actions

- internal organisational actions such as policy changes, paperwork or quality assurance audits

- financial and resource decisions

- the expectations and requirements of visitors to the service.

It is not that external factors are problematic in and of themselves. In fact, many of them are intended to have a positive impact on quality. Instead, this feature illustrates that it is the way in which these external factors are managed by the organisation that will determine whether they have a positive or detrimental effect on the care experiences of those receiving support. This means that both the external factors (e.g. a regulation inspector), and those responsible for acting on those factors within an organisation (e.g. a senior manager) must reflect and ensure that the impact of those external factors is positive on the experiences of those receiving care. Simply being designed with good intentions does not guarantee a measure will have a positive impact; the manner in which it is presented and implemented also matters. In positive care cultures, management in organisations actively consider the impact of measures from the point of view of front-line staff and those they support. They act as an intermediary between the external factor and the front line. They do this by absorbing the impact into their own roles or helping to translate the external factor's requirements into something that makes sense for staff in relation to people's care and well-being.

A practical example of mediation by management: Catherine's stay in hospital

Catherine is living with dementia and has been transferred to Ward B to recover from a broken hip. She has arrived with notes from Ward A that highlight a number of challenges. Catherine had fallen out of bed twice because of her desire to get up and walk despite her broken hip. She also continuously cries out for her husband, disturbing other patients. Her husband has become very distressed when asked to leave at the end of visiting time.

The senior sister on Ward B undertakes to meet with Catherine's husband to discuss her care. She feels that a change from the normal routine in the hospital may be beneficial. She manages to utilise a single room that is usually used for patients who require barrier nursing. She arranges for Catherine's husband to stay with Catherine around the clock, as this is what he would like. The sister discusses it with staff and writes in Catherine's notes, outlining why this is necessary. She makes a record on her audit form, anticipating that the ward may 'fail' on the monitoring visit due to non-compliance with visitor and bed allocation policy. She also leaves a copy for staff to give out when the monitoring assessment takes place.

She introduces a simple daily record sheet for staff to note the time they spend supporting Catherine (or her husband) and to keep a note of her distress levels. She helps staff to understand that it is needed so that they can see the impact of this change on staff time and on Catherine's well-being. As a result, Catherine's physical and emotional well-being improve significantly during her time on Ward B, as her husband is always by her side, relaxing her, supporting her to eat and preventing any falls. This means she is discharged much earlier than expected. Her husband is so pleased that he writes to the ward staff, the Trust Board and the local newspaper praising the care provided.

The actions here show that the sister on Ward B considered the impact of external pressures caused by (well-intentioned) hospital policy, and regulation has helped to improve Catherine's well-being and the resources of the hospital by hastening her recovery. She actively absorbed some of these pressures by anticipating the potential outcome of the monitoring visit and has helped staff to respond to some of them by demonstrating how it will improve Catherine's care. It is easy to see how, without such action, Catherine's recovery could be compromised and delayed because front-line staff are forced to take on the pressures of external factors of such policy compliance and feel compelled to ensure that their monitoring visit is a success. This is precisely what happened on Ward A: Catherine suffered because external pressures of policy compliance, visitor management and monitoring were transferred directly to staff, rather than being mediated by the ward sister.

This scenario also highlights another important feature necessary to create a positive care culture: those responsible for the external factors must allow and enable managers to take this mediating action and support an approach that considers the impact of any measure on front-line care delivery. Whether a regulator, safeguarding officer, internal auditor, quality assurance manager or visitor to a service, we have to understand that good intentions alone are not sufficient. We have to consider the impact they may have on the ground and work together with managers and staff in the organisation to make sure it has a positive rather than negative effect. This requires us to be critically reflective of our own practice and open to feedback from those working on the front line and those receiving care and support. What if the line manager of Ward B's sister is not understanding of the 'failed' monitoring report? What if the Trust Board fails to adapt its policies and procedures to suit patients like Catherine? Catherine and others like her will continue to be failed, despite everyone's good, 'quality improvement' intentions.

These values work together to create a virtuous circle of care

The four features outlined above are crucial for creating and sustaining a positive care culture in an organisation, which will help develop and maintain front-line action that promotes positive care experiences for people living with dementia and other complex needs. They interact with each other and all, therefore, are important. Measures to improve an organisation's culture need to take into account all four aspects, rather than focusing on one or another. This is because the four features described above can either create a virtuous or a vicious circle. Efforts to change culture can be reinforced when considered together or undermined when one or more features are neglected.

For example, an organisation may invest effort to develop a shared purpose and practical understanding of what person-centred care means for their patients, residents or service users. This could be done in any number of ways, such as training of staff, life story work with people living with dementia or changing paperwork, management approaches or recruitment etc. However, if consideration is not also given to how to empower staff to act on their understanding then they may be unable to make that practical understanding actually happen on the ground. If consideration is not also given to the effects of external pressures and how they can be mediated then the practical person-centred vision may be trumped on the ground by the need to demonstrate compliance with regulation or restricted by resource pressures. If consideration is not also given to creating a connectedness between everyone involved in that community then the practical vision of person-centred care breaks down, because people in the community may be working at cross purposes. Alternatively, considering all four elements means a practical vision of person-centred care is reinforced by a connected community because members of that community are actively involved in making it happen, highlighting and solving problems in achieving it. Empowered staff are able to enhance that community and vision in their daily actions, and external factors can be employed to supplement action on the ground rather than contradict it.

The norms of care behaviour

A further three features of a positive organisational culture are also very important. They are facilitated by the aspects highlighted above and, when they are seen regularly on the ground, they help to reinforce and sustain such positive values. They relate specifically to the 'norms of care' that can be observed and should be encouraged within front-line care. 'Norms' are the behaviours and actions that occur 'as normal'. They are what we would expect to see in all but the most exceptional situations. In fact, in a truly person-centred culture they may be so normal that they are done without conscious thought; *not* to do them would be seen as so unusual and strange that it would stand out and merit challenge and question. The norms of care here are most frequently seen within the actions and interactions of front-line caregivers and the people they are supporting, but it is important to remember that the elements outlined above are essential in allowing and encouraging them to happen.

Feature 5: Ongoing and gradual change for the benefit of people receiving care

We constantly look to make life better.

An openness and acceptance of the need for change is essential in creating a positive care culture. This is simply because people's needs, wants and goals change throughout their lives and on a moment-to-moment basis. This does not stop when someone has dementia and is in need of support from others. In fact, it becomes more important, because the effects of the dementia itself can have such a variable impact from day to day. This means that, if we want to provide truly person-centred care, openness and responsiveness to change need to be demonstrated and enabled on the front line. Change that is for the benefit of a person should be seen and acted on as a necessary and normal thing. However, successful cultures that create positive experiences whilst recognising this need for change also demonstrate a thoughtful approach to why and how that change is carried out. The goal (person-oriented rather than task-oriented) and the management of that change (gradual and ongoing rather than sudden) are crucial. Without this thoughtful approach, change is destabilising and will thus be problematic.

A positive care culture will expect and accept frequent change in the day-to-day routines, events and occurrences for each of the people it supports. Front-line staff will expect, and be supported, to facilitate that change. The changes that occur (or do not occur) each day will be understood and justified through the positive effects (both immediate and long term) they have on those receiving support. If change is not occurring, or is occurring to the detriment of a person, then it is questioned, reflected upon and altered if needs be. All change, whether small daily changes or large-scale organisational changes, need to be approached in the same gradual and person-oriented way in order to ensure a positive impact on the organisational culture.

Feature 6: Using the environment for the benefit of people receiving care

We help people enjoy the places where they spend time.

In a positive organisational culture, the immediate environment in which care and support takes place, whether a care home, hospital ward, GP surgery or person's own home, is constantly reflected upon by front-line staff to ensure it is as helpful as possible for the person living with dementia. This requires front-line staff to consider and act upon the appearance, noise, temperature, smell and usual routines of the environment. Whilst good, dementia-friendly design is helpful with this aspect, it is important to note that reflection on that environment is important whether the building is purpose built or not. It is what front-line staff are able to do with the environment that matters most. Each environment will come with its own advantages and limitations, but a positive culture encourages and facilitates creativity and flexibility in the environment.

A positive care culture will expect and accept that the environment needs to be as helpful (or made as helpful) as possible for the person living with dementia. Therefore it will encourage changes to the physical environment and what it is used for, in response to people's needs. In a positive culture it is normal to see front-line staff adapting the environment: chairs are moved, announcements are tailored to how a person best communicates, lighting is made brighter or darker and thought is given to whether a person is too warm or cold or whether they are distracted by background noise. All aspects of the environment whether temporary occurrences or long-term organisational decision-making are reflected and acted upon in relation to the effect on people living in or using the environment and those who are working with them.

Feature 7: Meaningful engagement and activity are integral to providing care and support

We help people to enjoy life in a way that fulfils them every day.

A positive care culture is also marked by the extent to which meaningful engagement with individuals and efforts to occupy and provide activity are integrated into the daily care, support and work of the service. This requires that engagement with people that is meaningful to them (whether through conversation, company or physical touch) is viewed as of equal importance to necessary physical tasks. It also requires that the need for meaningful occupation and prevention of boredom is understood as essential to a person's well-being and given equal weight to their physical well-being.

A positive care culture will expect and accept that meaningful engagement and activity are seen as often as physical aspects of care and support. It should be normal to see front-line staff sitting and chatting with people, and these interactions are not isolated to the completion of certain tasks or outcomes. It should be normal to see staff adapting their communication and approach to each person, whether by raising or lowering their voice or moving from behind the reception desk to show someone to their seat in the waiting room. It is normal to see items given to a person to engage with, meaningful music played, a person accompanying staff as they undertake their work or someone taking part in tasks or hobbies in a way adapted to their physical and cognitive abilities. Questions are asked when someone is not talked to, smiled at or occupied. Again, as well as being seen in day-to-day actions, organisational decisions need to consider and enable these features, whether through determining staffing levels, job descriptions or resources available.

The norms of care working together

As with the other four features, each of these aspects is as important as the other. You cannot have one without the other and so to focus efforts only on one feature without considering the others will undermine efforts.

A practical example of the three norms of care: Samira's good day

Imagine the care home where Samira lives. Staff at the home understand that changing what they do each day is important if it will benefit the residents, so they are always on the lookout for things that could be done better. When they notice that Samira is more restless than usual, they take a moment to think about why, and notice that the lounge where she is sitting is quite noisy as several residents are chatting to each other and the radio is on.

They talk to Samira to see if anything else is wrong and decide to see if she would be happier sitting somewhere quieter. However, they also know she does not like to be alone, so they ask the receptionist if she can sit in the foyer, as it is quieter but she will still have company. The receptionist moves her own chair so that Samira can sit with her behind the desk and she gives Samira a magazine to hold and talks to her about some of the pictures in the magazine at the same time as carrying on her work as best she can. She fetches an extra blanket for Samira when several people go in and out of the front door and let cold air in. When the deputy manager walks through to make a cup of tea she offers to get one for the receptionist and Samira so they can continue to sit and chat.

In this scenario, change, constant reflection on the environment and thoughtfulness about how best to engage with and occupy Samira are all absolutely necessary. Without all of them Samira is likely to experience ill-being either because change is difficult and resisted (feature 5), staff are not aware of the impact of the environment on Samira (feature 6) or they do not consider her need to be engaged with in a way that makes sense to her (feature 7).

In addition, you can see how the four previous elements also matter here: the home's staff are responsible and free to act to support Samira in the way they think best (feature 3), and everyone has a shared understanding of what being person-centred means for Samira in that moment (feature 1). The connectedness of the community means the receptionist understands how to help Samira as well as the staff (feature 2) and the deputy manager understands that the receptionist might be delayed in replying to emails, as she is busy chatting with Samira (feature 4).

Conclusion

Place the healthiest of plants in poor soil and it will struggle to thrive. A plant that is struggling needs the best possible quality of soil if it is to recover and continue to thrive. Alternatively, create a healthy soil and you will be surprised at the quality and diversity of plants that will grow. This is a good metaphor for thinking about care culture. Whether you are a person living with dementia, their partner, family, care worker, manager or a professional, your feelings and behaviour will be influenced by care culture. Moreover, dementia challenges a person and their relationships in the same way that any change, crisis or unhappy event can do. The culture needs to be strong to support these day-to-day crises, just as plants need to be well rooted to survive bad weather.

This book is designed to help you think about all the things that are important in implementing person-centred care. Aspects of culture and its influence, whether in society or through specific organisational dynamics, are highlighted throughout so that you can understand the powerful effect culture has on individuals and the ways in which they work with or live in a community with a person living with dementia. Whilst changing culture may feel as if it is an unassailable mountain, each of us can take small steps, and help others to take small steps, to climb it.

3

Valuing People

Element 1 of person-centred care is valuing people

Valuing people living with dementia and those who care for them: promoting citizenship rights and entitlements regardless of age or cognitive impairment, and rooting out discriminatory practice.

Key indicators of valuing

- **Vision**: Does everyone know what we stand for and share the vision?

- **Human resources**: Are systems in place to ensure staff know that they are valued as a precious resource?

- **Management ethos**: Are management practices empowering staff delivering direct care to ensure care is person-centred?

- **Training and staff development**: Are there systems in place to support the development of a workforce skilled in person-centred dementia care? Do staff know that supporting people living with dementia is treated as skilled and important work?

- **Service environments**: Are there supportive and inclusive physical and social environments for people living with cognitive disability? Do our places help people?

- **Quality assurance**: Are Continuous Quality Improvement mechanisms in place that are driven by knowing and acting upon needs and concerns of people with dementia and their supporters? Do we strive to get better all the time?

People with dementia are part of every community in society. They are not confined to some distant place away from the rest of humanity. The stigma that surrounds dementia, however, means that the problems we all face when living with dementia, or caring for others with dementia, are often not talked about. People living with dementia and those who care for them can become increasingly isolated, particularly as disabilities increase. We are, however, all citizens with all the rights that citizenship brings. We are also all human beings who depend on each other for love. People living with dementia are no less entitled to human rights or less in need of love.

The influence of society on care

Prevailing societal norms, values and attitudes operate in similar ways to the organisational culture of a care home or hospital, as discussed in Chapter 2. They govern what is acceptable or unacceptable to say, do and think in relation to people living with dementia or supporting someone living with dementia. Crucially, they influence us in unseen and unconscious ways – creating underlying assumptions and habits of thinking, feeling and responding to the day-to-day situations and circumstances we encounter.

Their unacknowledged and unquestioned influence is precisely their power. Those who do question them are viewed as eccentric at best and troublemakers at worst. However, change is only achieved by asking the seemingly eccentric question. If we never question why things are done in a certain way then nothing will ever change.

Services for people with dementia exist within society, and those providing these services are subject to the same prejudice as the rest of society. Within care services for people who are elderly, or who have mental health problems, those who have dementia often appear to be subject to even further prejudice. This discrimination is evident in service provision, resource allocation, research funding, media coverage, policy priorities and the professional training, status and pay of care workers.

Dementia is the most feared aspect of ageing (Alzheimer's Socity 2007). It is misunderstood by many, including those within the caring professions. Within western philosophy, the question of what it is that defines a living creature as a 'person' has received considerable attention. Some philosophers see the definition of person as being dependent on consciousness of thought (being able to think about yourself thinking) and continuity of memory (being able to know your continuous life story). Using this definition would mean that an individual with dementia would not be seen as the same 'person' as their dementia progressed, because their continuous memory of themselves would change. At the most disabling stages of dementia, when consciousness of thinking is no longer evident, then 'the person' would cease to exist. Using this definition, as dementia destroys the brain, it also destroys the person. This fits well with the view of dementia propounded in the media as a living death.

Our dementia-ist society, although improving, still frequently demonstrates that it that does not understand or accommodate people living with dementia and, in many situations, does not even attempt to try to do so. People continue to experience exclusion, discriminatory attitudes and isolation because others see the condition, label or unusual behaviour rather than seeing a person and member of the community, worthy of equal respect and understanding. This is perhaps not surprising, given that many would argue that our society still has a long way to go in properly integrating and involving people living with other physical or intellectual disabilities, evidences substantial ageism and struggles to accept and accommodate people of different races, faiths and sexualities. However, the challenges inherent to transforming cultural values that may contribute to discrimination and excess disability for people living with dementia should not deter us from attempting to transform them! In fact, the growing number of people living with the condition and the increased likelihood that we will be touched by it should spur us on.

Some countries have developed *dementia-friendly communities* programmes. People living with dementia want to remain independent for as long as possible and to have choice and control over their lives through all stages of dementia. The dementia-friendly communities programme improves awareness and understanding so that people can continue to enjoy the same facilities as everyone else, such as going to the shops, spending time with friends and family and using financial services. Alongside this work at community level, organisations from different sectors, such as banking, retail, transport and the fire and police services, are working together to help make their own sectors more dementia-friendly through activities such as improving awareness of dementia, training for staff and changes to their business processes.

Changing values is a slow process, but it is one that occurs with pressure from both the top and the bottom. Policies, politicians and local leaders matter and can drive positive change, but so can small, everyday acts. In fact, those everyday acts are often what help to highlight the difficulties and illuminate the ways in which things could be done differently. It is about ensuring that each and every one of us considers the needs of people living with dementia when setting up our services, taking part in our hobbies, doing our jobs, running our businesses or going about our daily lives in our community.

Do we display patience when the person in front of us in the queue struggles with the self-service checkout tills? Does the bank offer a way to retain independent access to money even though someone may not be able to remember a PIN? Does the local walking or fitness group, pub or cinema encourage people living with dementia to join in, actively making them welcome and accepted? Are the local police community support officers aware of how dementia may affect a person and those supporting them? Are our schools equipped to help children and young people to understand dementia and receive support when it affects their families? These are all questions we need to answer and encourage others to answer as well.

Changing landscapes

In many post-industrial societies there are increasingly dispersed family networks and complicated family structures. Many countries are increasingly multicultural, with many older people ageing in a second homeland. Moreover, societal views and cultural values on issues such as gender equality and sexual orientation have changed drastically between (and sometimes within) generations. Providing good transcultural, multicultural and genuinely inclusive care across generational boundaries is not easy. Increasingly, people find themselves being cared for by professionals and care workers who come from a different cultural background, with all the associated differences in values, norms and terms of reference than themselves. The shifting age demographics mean that there are fewer young people in society and an increasing number living into very old age.

The power of the words we use

Language is particularly important because it has a highly influential, although often unnoticed, effect. Words are not simply a way to communicate factual information to other people, but they also transmit *meaning*. When we do not reflect upon the underlying messages our choice of words may communicate, we can continue to send meanings and values that are unhelpful, by reinforcing stereotypes, perpetuating misunderstandings or objectifying and labelling a person or their situation. Considering the impact of language is also important because it is something that anyone, anywhere and in any position can influence. It is about reflecting on and changing the choices we as individuals make. We have the power to use language, which in turn can have an unintentional impact on others, for better or worse.

> Think about the type of language we commonly hear about dementia: 'time bomb', 'epidemic', 'burden', 'suffering'. Now imagine that you or someone close to you has just received a diagnosis of dementia. What images and underlying messages do those words send to you? Do they make you feel optimistic, hopeful, like there may be a light at the end of the tunnel? Or do they make you feel dispirited, demotivated, and overwhelmed? How might those feelings influence the way we think and behave towards people we encounter?

Considering the language that we use is not about putting a positive spin on things or pretending a situation is different to reality, but it is about being aware of the impact that words have, whether in conversation with a colleague or neighbour or through a newspaper or television report. Mrs Jones may well feel that she *suffers* through having dementia and her experience is hers and hers alone to describe. However, if we are to interact with Mrs Jones in whatever capacity, if we want to maximise her well-being despite her dementia, if we want her partner to know that we see her, not just her condition and if we want her neighbours to see her too, then the words we choose matter. Is Mrs Jones a 'dementia sufferer' to us, or is she 'living with dementia'?

If Mrs Jones is living with dementia, then we are more likely to feel that our responsibility is about helping Mrs Jones to *live* with her dementia – to get around the difficulties that dementia might bring. However, if Mrs Jones is a dementia sufferer, then we may get the message that this will be burdensome for us, that our responsibility is, at best, to put up with her dementia. Somewhere, in the use of this phrase, Mrs Jones herself has been lost. This is the case, whether we are Mrs Jones's nurse, neighbour or a cashier in her local supermarket.

Valuing personhood

Considering language and its common uses in relation to dementia helps to highlight another area of the culture that forms that soil in which we all grow: what is valued and devalued in and by our society and communities. Values underpin our behaviour by determining what is seen as normal, acceptable or encouraged within society. In short, they show us what is *valuable* to us, and therefore what we should treat as valuable. When talking to people living with dementia and those who support them (whether informally as family members or friends, or formally in professional roles) about their experiences, it is clear that we still live in a society that is dementia-ist.

Historically, and still today, people living with dementia have been treated as if they are non-persons. Once people have the label of dementia, it is assumed that people can no longer speak on their own behalf. This has been vigorously challenged in recent years. As dementia progresses, however, it can bring high levels of dependency.

It can become increasingly difficult to recognise the personhood behind the label.

Hughes (2001, 2011) provides a philosophical argument for defining a person as a 'situated-embodied-agent' rather than relying on consciousness of thought for the definition. Defining the concept of person like this means that we should aspire to treat people with dementia at all stages of their disability in the way in which all people would wish to be treated. Similarly, Kitwood (1993a) described the person with dementia as:

> a person in the fullest sense: he or she is still an agent, one who can make things happen in the world, a sentient, relational and historical being. (p.541)

In Kitwood's writing, the ethical standing of people with dementia was discussed in terms of personhood:

> Personhood…carries essentially ethical connotations: to be a person is to have a certain status, to be worthy of respect. (Kitwood and Bredin 1992b, p.275)

Likewise, John Bond (2001) described personhood as:

> all individuals are unique and have an absolute value… individuals do not function in isolation, they also have relationships with others; all human life is interconnected and interdependent. (p.47)

The lack of status and value that is attached to people with dementia also extends to those who want to look after their family members with dementia and those whose employment involves caring. Giving up paid employment to care for an elderly parent with dementia is not valued by society as much as staying at home to look after a terminally ill child. Likewise, the status afforded to a nurse working in a children's special care unit is much higher than the status of a nurse working in a care home.

Valuing the most vulnerable

On first contact, the moral and ethical basis for person-centred care is rather like 'mom and apple pie'. In this day and age, how could anyone disagree that treating people struggling to live with dementia as whole human beings is the right and civilised way to respond? However, a cursory look around service provision, or a discussion with people with dementia and their families, suggests that people with dementia are not valued by society and the care they receive is not based on trust, respect and dignity. Conversations with dedicated care workers will typically yield the phrase: 'I'm just a care worker', reflecting an internalisation of the unjustified disparagement and dismissal of that role so often seen and heard.

Person-centred care is not generally the stuff of headline news. It will not attract votes. Occasionally, scandals hit the media but they usually focus on issues of physical abuse or malnourishment. These episodes are dreadful but not commonplace. Rather, most poor-quality care and neglect that is experienced by people living with dementia is psychological rather than physical. Incomplete assessments, no one contacting you when they promised, feeling deceived, the withholding of information, the over-prescribing of drugs that you do not need and the under-prescribing of ones that you do. Lack of privacy, indignity, insensitivity, disrespect, stigmatisation, disempowerment and boredom are all very familiar features to service users and their families. The erosion of human and legal rights, and the overwhelming feeling that nothing personal is sacred, are still the day-to-day experiences of people with dementia and their families.

The personal is the political

Where does the will to provide person-centred care come from? Where do the champions and leaders of this cause come from? In the earlier section we saw that it is unlikely to be led at a government level. It is evident that things are changing, however. The rights of people with dementia are certainly more recognised than they were even five years ago.

In part, this is due to people with dementia speaking out for themselves. The practice of including people with dementia directly in the organisation of the Alzheimer's Society and other Alzheimer's Associations, and having people with dementia speak at national and international conferences, gives a very powerful message about the value of people with dementia in setting the agenda. However, those who are in long-term care are often too impaired and demoralised to be politically active. There are many excellent leaders in the dementia care field who also have the experience of being a family carer.

> The question remains as to how we can change the face of long-term care for people with dementia to ensure it is person-centred. Where is the leadership for this?
> The answer, gentle reader, is that it comes from you.

In many respects, it is surprising that a lot of services for people with dementia manage to operate in a way that *is* valuing of people with dementia. Fortunately, there have always been a good number of people who have operated with compassion and insight in their human relationships, even before we had any literature on person-centred care. There is a strong desire on an individual level from many people to provide health and social care that enables people to live their lives to the full. Sometimes this desire comes from family experience. Often it comes from a powerful drive for social justice and inclusion.

However, so often these positive experiences in health and care services can be traced to the dedication and resources of individuals investing personal time, money and physical and emotional energy to achieve what they know to be right for the people they support, rather than tracked to any systematic (whether societal or organisational) source. These individuals often find themselves to be swimming against a tide of indifference, which, over time, will erode the passion and motivation of all but the most exceptional individuals.

Being proactive in promoting the rights of people living with dementia has to be part of the definition of person-centred care. Unless we promote the value of people's lives then we collude with the message that the lives of those with dementia do not matter. Care practitioners need to be clear that caring for people with advanced dementia and co-morbidities is a skilled area of work that cannot be done successfully on the cheap by staff with no training. If we fail to do this then we are devaluing the lives of those we care for. If we devalue a person then this is not person-centred care.

Organisations that value people

If we encourage individual dementia care practitioners to adopt a person-centred approach without addressing the larger organisational context, we are setting them up to fail. The practice of caring for very vulnerable people with dementia in large groups with low staffing levels can place care workers in an intolerable bind when trying to provide person-centred care. How to balance the needs of one individual who requires lots of attention against the needs of the wider group, who may be equally needy but make less show of it, is one that faces dementia care practitioners, day in, day out. The previous chapters detailed how significant an organisational culture is in determining the experiences of people living with dementia. Creating an organisation that values people means addressing the aspects of that culture that influence what and who is valued and considering the variety of ways in which that value can be achieved.

Without acknowledgement of its importance and constant effort to affect that culture through factors such as continuous quality management, training and daily support for direct care staff, even workers with good hearts can begin to think that neglectful practice is acceptable and normalise poor standards of care. Moreover, for vulnerable, low-paid staff, dependent on their employer to ensure their bills are paid, there can appear little choice but to continue carrying out poor practice even if one's head and heart knows that it is abusive. If staff's attempts to raise concerns go unheard then this feeling of powerlessness worsens and those who can afford to leave their employ will do so, leaving only those who do not recognise abuse and neglect or who are unable to challenge it.

This further embeds a poor culture of care. When circumstances of poor culture develop, the situation can escalate quickly, with services developing a poor reputation, making recruitment difficult. This results in a very unstable, high-stress environment for both staff and residents. This environment is then supporting a highly vulnerable group of people for whom instability and stress are toxic.

If an organisation is to deliver person-centred care in anything but a non-tokenistic manner, the rights of all people regardless of age and cognitive ability have to be driven from all directions and be led from the top levels of organisations. The person-centred approach is an ethical code that encompasses all relationships. This includes not just people with dementia but also those of us who work in this area and those who are family carers. It is a code that values all people as unique individuals, seeks authentic connections and tries to see things from the viewpoint of the other and recognises the interdependence of us all. Organisations that adopt a person-centred approach to care also recognise the need to work by the same set of principles with their staff.

Rather than seeing people with dementia as the ones having problems and those who are caring as having none, Kitwood suggested that many of the problems experienced in dementia care are interpersonal. They occur in the communication. He suggests we need to view the relationships between 'carers' and 'cared for' as psychotherapeutic relationships and, in this respect, just as in psychotherapeutic work, the helpers need to be aware of their own issues around caring for others. In person-centred care, the relationships between all people in the care environment should be nurtured:

> I believe that people with dementia are making an important journey from cognition, through emotion, into spirit. I've begun to realise what really remains throughout this journey is what is really important, and what disappears is what is not important. I think that if society could appreciate this, then people with dementia would be respected and treasured. (Bryden 2005, p.159)

Valuing people is at the heart of person-centred care. If this element of the definition is not made explicit in statements, training, staff selection, standards, policies and procedures, and if its connection with the overall culture is not considered, then services will not maintain a person-centred approach for long.

Putting valuing into practice

The indicators in the valuing people element of VIPS primarily need to be led by those managing the health or social care organisation. These indicators are about the organisational vision and leadership and how these are operationalised in practice. Crucially, these need to be considered as part of a continual process of reflection and renewal, in which individual aspects of person-centred care interact with the culture already in existence to enhance or detract from actual experiences on the ground. The VIPS Framework is not about taking a single action to tick a box, such as writing a policy or organising training. Instead it is about exploring the experiences of those receiving and delivering support, considering how each of these indicators might be impacting (positively or negatively) on those experiences and, most importantly, acting to maintain or change that impact.

This can feel as if it is a never-ending battle! As managers and leaders of organisations providing care and support, it sometimes feels that all we can do is struggle to find the resources to meet minimum standards of basic physical care. Working within cash constraints, dealing with staff shortages and being the repository for everyone's complaints and guilt grind managers down over time. They can diminish the personhood of those in leadership positions, which means that those of us who are responsible for setting the value base for an organisation often feel devalued ourselves.

Providing person-centred care that values all people is in itself a journey. The fact that you are reading this book means that you have already started travelling. What follows are a series of questions to help you reflect on where you are in terms of the valuing people aspect of person-centred care and think about what you need to consider to improve and sustain a positive care culture in this regard.

We outline why each question is important in providing person-centred care, what evidence an organisation or provider might look for in order to answer the questions posed and what elements of positive care culture it is worth considering if you wish to address and improve this aspect of person-centred care.

1. Vision: Does everyone know what we stand for and share the vision?

An organisation's mission statement spells out its reason for being and its purpose. Valuing people has to begin at the top and it has to begin with a purposeful intent. Valuing the equality of all regardless of age and cognitive disability is a challenge that is difficult to achieve. It is impossible to achieve fully unless those at board or trustee level take it as underpinning all their decisions. Agreeing this in its vision or mission statement means that the organisation is making public its policy of promoting the rights of people with dementia.

Vision is important for organisational culture because it sets the tone and direction of everything the organisation does. Crucially, in order really to ensure that a vision or mission statement is affecting culture positively, you need to think about how that vision is actually understood and enacted in practical terms. Feature 1 of positive care cultures was that *we all work together to deliver the best care*, and this emphasises the importance of vision and its practical application. Can the mission statement for the service easily be translated into what it might mean for Person X? Does staff member Y know what practical things they can do within their work role to make that vision happen? Does everyone share understanding of what this vision means in practice or do different people hold different interpretations?

Talking about, creating and reviewing the vision with everyone involved in the service can help to ensure that *we all matter to each other*. This connectedness in turn helps everyone to play their part in making the vision happen. A leadership that *protects front-line service delivery* helps ensure that the vision is practically achieved for people in action rather than words. Where there is potential conflict between external requirements and achieving the vision on the ground, the organisation (through the owner, director or senior managers) needs to take responsibility for managing and resolving that conflict, rather than leaving front-line staff to deal with the consequences.

Developing a mission statement is an exercise in setting the value base of an organisation. It has to involve all the key stakeholders if it is to be owned and abided by. Management textbooks devote significant space to advice on developing mission statements.

Written material about the service should be provided in a way that is accessible to all people who come into contact with the service. This includes a vision statement about people being supported by the service regardless of their age or level of cognitive ability, and how this is achieved. This information should also be available in spoken and other formats where appropriate. This purpose should be clear to all members of staff at all levels from direct care to board level. It should be clear to service users, their families and all who come into contact with the service.

In the CHOICE project, this care home manager described her own organisation's vision for person-centred care and highlighted the need constantly to strive toward it lest progress be lost:

> We should be looking at what the resident wants and trying to achieve that wherever we possibly can, rather than looking at what the staff want and working to what the staff find easiest, although…it will always revert, however much they understand person-centred care, person-centred care always reverts to yourself, doesn't it? But I think that's our ethos.

This practical approach of 'what the resident wants' was evident throughout the work of the home every day. This showed not only in the care experiences of residents but also in the attitudes of staff. When various members of staff were asked what advice they would first give to a new member of staff, they all replied along similar lines: 'Just get to know your residents.'

Part 2 of this book (page 183) has questions to help you think about your organisation's performance on this indicator.

---

2. Human resources: Are systems in place to ensure staff know that they are valued as a precious resource?

If an organisation values people for their inherent worth as human beings then it will seek to fight discrimination of all sorts. Are people from all walks of life welcome? This is part of person-centred care for staff. If the staff feel valued then they in turn are likely to value those they care for. This should be reflected in practices that affect recruitment, promotion, pay and conditions, and that reward skills and expertise in person-centred care.

If staff are to see communication, integrity and nurturing as important in their work with people with dementia then this should be their experience of how the organisation relates to them as workers. Is there a recognition of the importance of building teams that work well together and are united in their purpose? Teams that see value in working together are more likely to promote a sense of shared community with all the service users in their facility, with less risk of scapegoating those people who do not fit in easily. Is there a whistle-blowing policy? How is sickness managed? What sort of induction, appraisal and reward systems exist? What are the terms and conditions of employment?

How is workplace stress managed? Providing person-centred dementia care is emotionally labour intensive; how is it identified when a team is in need of extra support? What form does extra support take? How is it accessed? How is it reviewed? Is there a system of debriefing and reflection following particularly stressful events?

Approaches to managing and supporting staff are important to culture because they are the way we lead by example and role model what person-centred approaches we wish to see in care delivery. *We empower and support front-line staff* was a central feature of a positive care culture. Without careful consideration of how management practices support (or fail to support) both the responsibility and autonomy of staff in their work, any positive aspects of culture will be patchy and unreliable. Crucially, this is not simply about formal approaches such as supervision and recruitment, but also about informal aspects of leadership, spread across a team rather than focused on one person in a hierarchical structure.

Human resource management is truly valuing when it reflects on the following: How does the way the management team communicate and interact with staff show that their need for practical and emotional support is recognised? Is the management team present, available and responsive to staff requests and encouraging of their input? Does the way in which staff are managed clearly define people's roles and responsibilities? Do staff experience management as consistent, fair and as having integrity?

Here are two contrasting case studies that show how interactions and approach to staff can treat them as a precious resource or result in a feeling of being devalued.

In this first example, the manager explains her approach to supporting staff, which was witnessed in action and mentioned frequently by staff as something that helped them and contributed to their commitment to their work and workplace:

> Here we do a lot of informal chat where people come in and sit and talk about issues. Because I have an open-door policy you see, and that saves a lot of hassle because everybody knows they can come and say and talk to me… It's important for the staff as well to know that they've got a platform that they can talk from as well.

However, in this second example, these two care workers talk about their organisation's approach:

> When it came to it and I went well what about [training she had been told would be available]: 'Well you can pay for it yourself.' …now, I'm sorry, but on a minimum wage of six pounds eighty I can't afford to take any courses whatsoever, I am only just getting by, and then it was, 'Oh well.'
>
> We do, like a very, very basic couple of hours on dementia. Anything else, you would have to go and do yourself and pay for it yourself, which I have done…but it's a hundred and fifty pounds, and some carers don't have that for these things, you know, courses and stuff like that.

Part 2 of this book (page 184) has questions to help you think about your organisation's performance on this indicator.

3. Management ethos: Are management practices empowering to staff delivering direct care to ensure care is person-centred?

Providing person-centred care for people with dementia often relies on taking advantage of opportunities as they occur. Staff who feel their ideas for good practice are met with enthusiasm are more likely to react positively to ideas and challenges from service users. If a 'can-do' culture exists for staff they are more likely to promote this with service users and families.

Markers of this might include clear avenues for communication that are used frequently between different levels of the organisation. How are decisions made and disseminated throughout the organisation? Staff who feel that they understand why decisions have been taken, and are knowledgeable about the process, are surely more likely to keep families and service users better informed in a way that deals with issues rather than apportions blame for bad decisions to the powers that be.

Is there a consultation process that is trusted throughout the organisation? Staff who feel that they have been consulted over practice are more likely to institute consultation practices with families and service users. Is there an 'open-door' management practice? Staff who feel that they can approach their managers if they have a problem that they cannot resolve, or an idea that will improve practice, are more likely to encourage and listen to ideas from families and service users. Is there delegation of resource management to the optimum level to provide person-centred care?

Without the ability to communicate effectively with each other, the basis for providing an adequate social environment is flawed. In the absence of good communication, paranoia, confusion and anxiety flourish. This is true both for staff teams and for people receiving support. How are matters communicated between members of staff? Is adequate time provided for handovers and communal problem-solving? Who talks to whom? What is the communication like within a shift? What is the communication like between front-line and senior staff? What is communication like between shifts, between night and day staff, between staff working in different sections of the same building? Is the communication two-way? Do people feel listened to and have the chance to have their say?

Management ethos highlights the importance of creating a culture in which *we empower and support front-line staff.* Day-to-day approaches to management, communication and problem-solving need to ensure that they are truly responsive and supportive of front-line staff in their daily work. They need to be in tune with what is really happening on the ground through the experience of those receiving support, rather than focused solely on restating what it 'should' be like. If something is not right on the ground, do management approaches focus on discovering why and supporting changes to happen?

A management ethos is truly valuing of people when management consider the norms of care and support they wish to see on the ground and reflect on the impact of their actions (and inaction) on achieving them in practice. Do they help enable these norms of care: *we constantly look to make things better for people, we help people to enjoy places where they spend time, we help people to be active in a way that fulfils them every day?*

There is also an implication here about the importance and influence of connectedness and community. The ethos of management can lead the way in ensuring that *we all matter to each other,* that everyone has a role to play in the 'community' of a service or organisation. Ensuring that people's experiences and ideas are listened and responded to provides a route for everyone to take part and see their impact on the community.

In this example, a resident's relative who also contributed to the care home's voluntary committee talks about the management ethos she has seen in practice – something she felt contributed to the high standard of care for residents:

I think they've got a very good team of management here. I think the way [manager and head of care] work, pull together, they care for the staff, they're very fair. I think that gels, it sets the tone, and they know exactly where they're going so that obviously is shown down to the staff, which of course is then shown out to the residents. So I think good strong management at the top. Enthusiastic, each goes beyond their call of duty. Because [manager] always says, 'They're my residents,' it's not just a job to her. And the same with [head of care], they want to be here and they exude such enthusiasm that I feel that is passed on to the staff. And because they then feel motivated, they've got someone they can go and talk to, and I think if the staff are satisfied then it's going to lead to happier residents isn't it?

As the manager explained herself:

I think you've got to be prepared to do that, you can't just sit in your office, you've got to be prepared to say 'Well I'll get the mop, I'll scrub,' you know. I go and do the gardening, I stick my dirty clothes on sometimes and I go 'Right I'm coming to sort this garden out,' and I'll go and do it. And it helps I think.

Part 2 of this book (page 185) has questions to help you think about your organisation's performance on this indicator.

4. Training and staff development: Are there systems in place to support the development of a workforce skilled in person-centred dementia care? Do staff know that supporting people living with dementia is treated as skilled and important work?

Maintaining person-centred care over time for people with dementia is not an easy or trivial process. Dementia services do not have a tradition of skilled care or the practices that are required to maintain it. Wages and status (and associated high turnover of staff) exacerbate the difficulties inherent in altering this state of affairs. There should be a recognition within a person-centred organisation that caring for people with dementia is skilled work that is emotionally and physically labour intensive. What is the training and education strategy? What is available at induction regarding working with people with dementia? How are training needs identified? What specialist courses are available? What is the level of expertise of more senior people?

How is learning supported in the workplace? Are there opportunities for reflective practice, supervision and mentoring? When individual practitioners or staff teams are feeling out of their depth working with a particular person or family, how is more expert help accessed?

Considering training and development practice in relation to organisational culture highlights something very important in making this aspect of valuing influential for person-centred care. Training and development need to be focused towards and evaluated against what they achieve on the ground. They need to be seen holistically and as part of a whole range of factors that affect care and support experiences, not the *only* solution. There can be a tendency for training to be identified as an easy remedy for less than positive care on the ground, without other aspects being considered.

Remember that positive care cultures require us to *empower and support front-line staff.* They also require that staff are enabled to *constantly look to make things better,* to *help people to enjoy the places where they spend time* and to *help people to be active in a way that fulfils them every day.* Organisations achieve training and development that is truly valuing of people when the training, needs analysis or development plan are accompanied by other, more subtle actions: How do management teams discover what prevents staff putting things into practice with service users? Are there opportunities to reflect on daily challenges and put increased knowledge into action? Are there highly skilled individuals available who are practically able to support and mentor others?

In this case study, the management had sought to introduce team leaders in some areas of the home units to help enhance person-centred care. They also used this as a way to develop staff skills, showing faith in one care worker who sought promotion (despite their initial doubts). This worker, turned out to be a fabulous and influential team leader in improving the well-being of residents.

As the head of care explained:

When she came into the interview she astounded us both, I think we both sat there like this [open mouthed] thinking, 'Well this isn't

> the person that we thought we knew.' And since she, like the first day in her new role, she's immediately, she's transformed. And I think it's because she's matured. She is only young, but she's sort of found her feet and found her place and has suddenly realised that, you know, what other people think, it doesn't matter if what you think is right, and that's what came over.

The manager too expressed the same desire to allow the staff member to develop:

> I didn't think [staff member], ...she'd been a mouse. I didn't think she'd cope at all. And then she was totally different in interview and I thought, 'I've got to give her a go from how she's come over in interview.' And again, it was that business of [her] saying, 'If I know I'm right, I will stand up to them,' and I thought 'Right, I'm going to let you try,' and she has – from the word go.

Part 2 of this book (page 186) has questions to help you think about your organisation's performance on this indicator.

5. Service environments: Are there supportive and inclusive physical and social environments for people living with cognitive disability? Do our places help people?

Once an organisation has taken on board the need to eradicate discriminatory practice against people with dementia, the next stage is to look at the active steps it takes to support people with dementia. If an organisation is able to give examples of providing individualised care, taking seriously the viewpoint of people with dementia and providing a supportive social psychology, as outlined in other chapters in this book, then it is likely it is serious about its commitment to anti-discriminatory practice.

Anti-discriminatory practice means that people with dementia have the same rights as everyone else. It does not mean that people with dementia do not need extra help in everyday life. For example, we would expect that those in wheelchairs to have a right to enter buildings, and we would provide elevators or ramps to help them achieve this. Likewise, we would expect that a person with dementia to have the right to find their way around the building with clear signage and way-finding markers.

At a corporate level, this means that there should be evidence that this is taken into consideration in design briefs for buildings and for fixtures and fittings. The general physical design should include features such as clear colours, way-finding memory markers, unambiguous surfaces to walk on, easy access to a safe outdoor environment, natural light, low numbers of blind corners, no obvious locked doors and unobtrusive use of technology maximised to provide a non-confusing and low anxiety-provoking physical environment. Many tools exist to help assess the dementia-friendly nature of building and design.

At a corporate level, there should also be recognition that all staff coming into contact with service users with dementia should understand some of the special needs around communication. Is it policy that all staff having direct service-user contact are aware of how to help someone with dementia feel at ease? Is this evidenced in staff induction and training? Many organisations have undertaken 'Dementia Friends' programmes to underline the importance of this for all staff.

The role of the service environment links directly to the 'norms of care' that are important for creating positive care cultures. Most importantly, they also demonstrate how critical it is to approach achieving person-centred care as an ongoing process, rather than a one-stop checklist approach. Nowadays we see a plethora of 'dementia-specialist' environments and equipment advertised, but by themselves they do not guarantee that people will experience their support positively. It is how these are then used in combination with people's needs and how changes and limitations are responded to that is significant. Organisations achieve service environments that are truly valuing of people with dementia when they are used in a way that *helps people to enjoy places where they spend time.* This requires that staff are able to *constantly look to make things better* and *help people to be active in a way that fulfils them every day.*

Being able to use the environments in a way that is valuing also requires that *leadership protects front-line service delivery* from external factors that may prevent this flexible use of the service environments. This requires both organisations and those outside of services, such as regulators, to understand and enable this to happen, particularly when conflicting issues such as freedom and safety come into play.

Here, two contrasting examples show how different organisational approaches lead to environments that can value people living there or devalue and disable them. First, a care worker talks about how they were encouraged to use all the spaces available in a (very old, institutional style building) to provide for people's differing needs:

> [I] set up two rooms, one in the small lounge and one in the main lounge, and the one in the main lounge is normally more sensory for the less able residents, and the one in the small lounge is for the residents that might be able to understand a [DVD], like the *Frozen Planet*, or the Hymns, or something in the small lounge, and then we can split the residents up based on their ability. And I say 'Oh I've set these up,' to the other carers, you know, 'Put so and so in there, and so and so in there, if they want to go in.'

However, in this case study, an organisational decision had resulted in an environment that was less supportive of residents, as these observational notes explain:

> I chat with the staff about the position of the 'cosy corner' [an area of seating down the end of a corridor that is not used by residents]. They explain that it used to be in the centre of the hall, residents really liked it as they could see everything that was going on. But the computer was installed there [by the organisation's IT department] for the carer's computerised records and it got very busy and 'caused an obstruction'. They said that since the cosy corner moved down to [the] end it is hardly used.

Part 2 of this book (page 187) has questions to help you think about your organisation's performance on this indicator.

6. Quality assurance: Are Continuous Quality Improvement mechanisms in place that are driven by knowing and acting upon needs and concerns of people with dementia and their supporters? Do we strive to get better all the time?

Knowing how service users feel about the service they receive on an ongoing basis is central to person-centred care. How does the organisation know and act upon the views of people receiving care and support? Does it undertake regular satisfaction surveys, interviews, focus groups, reference groups or observation of practice? Are the views of all service users regardless of level of cognitive impairment taken into account in this process or just the most vocal?

Involving service users and knowing their views is central to person-centred care – or any customer-care activity. In the dementia care field, this can take place through residents' groups, carers' groups, user forums and other ad hoc reference groups. How are these organised? How often do they occur? Whose responsibility are they? What happens to the views or decisions made at these meetings? Are they seen as central to the decision-making process or are they just an add-on? Moreover, how do we access the viewpoint of those who cannot take part or communicate easily?

Three features of positive cultures are significant if quality assurance in an organisation is to help provide services that are truly valuing of people living with dementia. Organisations in which *we all matter to each other* and in which *we all work together to deliver the best care* ensure that quality assurance is an ongoing and impactful process because everyone involved in the services has a role to play that is clearly understood in terms of achieving person-centred services for people. This means that people feel more confident and responsible for making comments, asking questions, suggesting changes and solving problems. Without consideration of these elements, quality assurance can exacerbate feelings of 'them and us' and be experienced as antagonistic or become more of a tokenistic effort, rather than something that results in positive change. If *we empower and support front-line staff* then staff will also be more likely to engage in processes of day-to-day quality assurance, because they are free to act on any issues and expected and supported to do so.

In this care home, quality assurance was recognised as something that needed to be employed every day, and the manager had altered the staff team set up so that team leaders could be responsible for this:

> I thought the only way we're going to get that implemented is if we do have team leaders to lead it, because the nurses are too busy doing the nurse bits. It's worked, so it's right. I mean I'll probably have to argue the toss at budget but I'll...argue that, because we can see what it's done...there's things happening and people are bobbing about, and those staff who are a bit slack are being, you know, I just, [a team leader] said last night 'You can't do that!' but nobody had noticed before.

This is in contrast to a different care home where more formal routines of quality management often had an opposite effect to their intention, as these observational notes show:

> A lady with a badge and a clipboard came along the corridor [the regional manager]. She talked to residents, talked to the carers who arrived with the tea trolley, she commented on the [cake] not going very quickly and the carers seemed a little defensive in their response, [saying] that they had only just started... I asked the regional manager how often she visited...and I felt quite uncomfortable that she stood leaning on the back of the sofa talking to me behind a resident's head. I wondered if the carers noticed this and thought it wasn't very person-centred.

Part 2 of this book (pages 188–189) has questions to help you think about your organisation's performance on this indicator.

Summary

The first aspect of person-centred care is about valuing people throughout the organisation. If staff do not feel valued by the organisation they work for then it is unlikely they will be able to sustain valuing and caring relationships with people with dementia over time. Valuing people can be seen in many organisational processes around communication, anti-discriminatory practice, human-resources management, training, operational management, consultation and quality management. The multiple ways in which we might seek to value people in our organisation need to be introduced, adapted and reviewed in ways that are mindful of the need positively to affect and use the organisational culture that exists. Merely doing something is not enough, we must continually think about how we do it and ensure that it sends the right message in reality as well as intention.

4

Individual Lives

Element 2 of person-centred care is recognising that all people are different

Recognising that people are individuals, appreciating that all people have a unique history and personality, physical and psychological strengths and needs, and social and economic resources, and that these will affect their response to dementia. Care and support needs to be tailored to this.

Key indicators of an individualised approach to care

- **Care and support plans**: Do our care and support plans promote individual identity showing that everyone is unique, with hopes, fears, strengths and needs?

- **Regular reviews**: Do we recognise and respond to change?

- **Personal possessions**: Do people have their favourite and important things around them? Do we know why they're meaningful for them?

- **Individual preferences**: Are a person's likes, dislikes, preferences and choices, listened to, known about and acted upon?

- **Life story**: Are a person's important relationships, significant life stories and key events known about and referenced in everyday activities?

- **Activity and occupation**: Is a person's day full of purpose and engagement with the world, regardless of their needs and abilities?

The most concrete expression of person-centred care, which sometimes becomes its whole definition, is about taking an individualised approach to assessing and meeting the needs of people with dementia. This element of the definition encompasses all those ways of working that consider people with all their individual strengths and vulnerabilities and sees their dementia as part of that picture rather than defining their identity. This approach has resonance with the work of Carl Rogers for whom each client was a unique and whole person.

Every person's experience of dementia is unique. It is shaped by the dementia itself and how that changes over time, but also the person's life history and personality play a part alongside family and community context. Individualised assessment, analysis and case management focus on this area of person-centred care. Understanding a person's lifestyle and preferences is crucial to providing person-centred care for people with dementia. Using positive memories can be helpful in improving self-esteem and to maintain an identity in the face of increasing confusion. Familiar touchstones of our cultural identity, our spirituality or religion, food, drinks and music are likely to have a calming effect. Vulnerability, anxiety and alienation are more likely to increase if those elements are missing.

It is often difficult to access this life-story information once dementia has progressed, although there are an increasing number of tools to help with this (e.g. Saunderson and Bailey 2013). It is better still for a person to make a record of important events, touchstones and preferences at an early stage following diagnosis so that this information is accessible to others when needed. This can include information about lifestyle preferences as well as advance decisions about end-of-life care. Many National Dementia Strategies advocate that citizens should have access to accurate diagnosis *at a time* in the disease process when it can be of most benefit to them. The term *timely diagnosis* is used to reflect this. The diagnosis can help people and their families make sense of what is happening and make lifestyle changes and plans for the future (Brooker *et al.* 2014).

As dementia progresses, it can be difficult for the person to remember important information and to tell others about this. This is true for information about health, preferences and wishes as well as the key stories of one's life and identity. The provision of easily accessible information, about the person's health and preferences as well as life stories, is helpful here.

Is individualised care the same as person-centred care?

One of the original drivers for developing the VIPS definition of person-centred care was to differentiate it from 'individualised' care. This was epitomised in the publication of the UK *National Service Framework for Older People* (DoH 2001) that interpreted person-centred care as having an individualised plan of care to meet individual needs to promote independence. If the intention is solely to look at a person's needs in the context of their being a patient or a resident then it is probably clearer to use the term 'individualised patient care' or 'individualised resident care'. In Germany, the term 'patientenzentriert' – 'patient centred' has existed for many years and is used with respect to care in hospitals. Likewise, the term 'patient-centred' is used frequently in the UK, the USA and Australia. Although this is clearly linked to the individualised care element of person-centred care, it provides a much narrower focus than person-centred care, in that the person can only express those individual needs that are covered by being a patient.

Personalisation, consumer-driven care and personal budgets are all important developments. They are potential means of putting people in the driving seat of achieving the care they want. However, these are ways of achieving individualised care programmes rather than being definitions in themselves of person-centred care. Although it is not possible to achieve person-centred care without taking an individualised approach, it is possible to achieve individualised care that is not person-centred. Inserting a problem focus into individualised care can make it difficult to continue to see the person as an individual in the round.

Those working in the care professions can become so conditioned by defining people they work with by their diagnostic group, problem type or service need, that they are at risk of overlooking the person behind the label. For example a person (who is a patient in a hospital) might be able to have an individualised plan of continence care but not be able to make a cup of tea, because the risk is too great for the hospital's insurers. The person in this context is defined by their status as a patient having continence needs, rather than an appreciation of their need to maintain a lifelong activity such as making tea. There is a danger that, by focusing only on individualised care, the person with dementia stays firmly hidden behind their disease label and person-centred care still does not occur.

Moreover, focusing only on individualised care rather than a truly person-centred approach leaves the impact of culture unacknowledged and untouched. It is the culture of a service or community, (its norms, rules and language played out day to day) that create the 'patient', 'resident' or 'client' as a distinct identity that is separate from those who provide support and those in the 'outside world'. This culturally given identity comes with a range of often unspoken expectations, assumptions and rules of behaviour that (deliberately or unintentionally) reinforce differences and affect the relationships that form between people receiving support, those providing it and others from outside the service or organisation.

By contrast, when considered in depth, person-centred care drives us to think about the ways in which each person's unique identity is affected, enhanced or challenged by the culture of our services, support or society and demands that we adapt. If our support and services are truly person-centred then the person should shape what the organisation does and says, rather than the organisation shaping and redefining the person to suit what is usually provided. Using individuals' unique identities and experiences as the basis for creating the support provided for them when they are living with dementia will require that our culture is reflective and adaptive to the differences within and between each person we encounter.

Individual lives make us who we are

Kitwood (1990a, 1990b) characterised dementia as a dialectical interplay between neurological impairment, the psychological make-up of the individual with dementia and the social context (social psychology) in which they find themselves. This later became the Enriched Model of dementia, incorporating the biological, the psychological and the social aspects of a care environment, which is summarised in Table 4.1.

The equation in Table 4.1 aids understanding of the unique position of each person with dementia. Every such person will have a different pattern of neurological impairment, a different health profile, a unique history and personality and a distinctive interplay of all these in the social aspects of their current situation. It is a person-centred model rather than a biological model and has many uses in assessment and care practice (for example May, Edwards and Brooker 2009). Some of the terms might sound a little dated now but the model has been used by many over the years as a means of understanding the experience of dementia in how it impacts on an individual's life.

Table 4.1 The Enriched Model of dementia

Dementia = NI + H + B + P + SP
NI = Neurological impairment
H = Health and physical fitness
B = Biography – life history
P = Personality
SP = Social psychology

Neurological impairment (NI)

There are many different types of dementia and these will impact on the brain in different ways over time. There is no one pattern of neurological impairment. However, in order to support an individual we have to understand the symptoms of cognitive impairment they are struggling with. The neurological impairment associated with dementia often (but not always) affects memory function, the ability to use and understand spoken and written language, the ability to carry out practical everyday tasks, the ability to perceive the world as others do and the ability to plan a course of action and to see things from other people's viewpoints. These impairments are quite subtle and easy to misunderstand at first, but become more obvious as the dementia progresses over time. Being aware of the manifestation of these impairments is a key element of good dementia care in enabling supporters to respond appropriately. The aim is to find a response that supports the person with dementia while not undermining their remaining abilities.

Common cognitive impairments in dementia, such as poor learning of new information, dysphasias, dsypraxias and visuo-perceptual deficits, mean that people with dementia will interpret their social and physical environments in a unique way. If these interpretations of the environment are not understood and compensated for then the person with dementia will experience excess disability. All too often, however, this is attributed to neurological impairment rather than as a function of an unsupportive care environment (Stokes 2000). Some of the behaviours that are sometimes labelled as 'challenging' or 'disturbed' are simply a result of the impairment that a person is dealing with. For example, a person may become very frightened of a dressing gown on the back of a bedroom door because their brain is misperceiving it as a stranger standing in the room. Removing the dressing gown may take away the 'hallucination' and avoid the person being labelled simply because of their neurological impairment.

It is important to recognise that individuals will still have many cognitive strengths that can be used to help them maintain independence in many areas of day-to-day life. For example, long-held skills such as cooking and housework may be relatively intact. Although the ability to plan a meal may be lost, the person may well be able to accomplish parts of the process – such as chopping vegetables – very well. Providing aids and adaptations (such as GPS systems or electronic reminders) to help people cope better with the impairments means that the disability is lessened. By understanding the neurological impairment profile we can optimise functioning and provide a rehabilitative enabling environment.

Health and physical fitness (H)

If a person has a label of dementia, there is a tendency for others to attribute any increase in confused behaviour to the dementia.

However, people living with dementia are also much more susceptible to acute confusional states and delirium arising from physical health problems such as urinary or chest infections, constipation, hormonal imbalances, dehydration, malnutrition, over-medication and sedation. This is compounded further by the fact that some people with dementia will not be able to give an accurate account of their symptoms because of their memory problems. For example, if a person with dementia is unable to remember that they have been experiencing chest pains, they are unlikely to seek help for their symptoms. Pain is very under-reported in dementia and there are a number of research studies that have demonstrated that simple pain relief can dramatically reduce so called 'challenging behaviour' (Husebo *et al.* 2011). People living with dementia may not complain of pain or say they are in pain when asked. However, changes in behaviour can indicate an underlying physical health problem. There are a number of well-validated pain assessment scales that are very useful in this respect. It is incumbent on those delivering care to be extra vigilant regarding changes in physical health status.

Biography or life history (B)

Everyone, regardless of cognitive ability, makes sense of what is happening to them in the here and now by reference to experiences they have had in the past. However, because of the neurological impairment, particularly in Alzheimer's-type dementia, the more recent past for people is often not laid down reliably within memory stores. People with dementia who are in a nursing home, for example, may have very little understanding of where they are. First, they may not remember anything about the admission process because of memory loss and, second, nursing homes do not relate to any past experiences they have.

Nonetheless, people will try to make sense of where they are. For example, for some, the nursing home may look rather like their former workplace or being in the GP surgery may feel as if they are sitting outside the head teacher's office. Knowledge of someone's life history may again help staff to understand so-called 'challenging behaviour'. For example, people who have held managerial positions during their working life may find it very confusing to be told what to do by a care worker who, in their eyes, is a junior employee, particularly if what they are being told to do relates to personal care activities. Likewise, if a person with dementia thinks that it is time to pick children up from school then they may become very angry when someone tells them it is not safe to leave the hospital ward.

Past experiences of institutional care are particularly important to know about. For example:

- A person who is the ex-head teacher of a school may wish to give direction and search through paperwork and timetables and may not take kindly to being told that they may not do so by someone they consider to be their junior staff or pupils.

- A person who has spent time in a children's home, prison, or refugee camp at an earlier time of their life may interpret particular staff actions in ways that use old memories of the past and act accordingly, such as by hiding food, keeping to rigid routines or avoiding certain spaces, people or situations.

Personality (P)

This refers to the totality of the strengths and vulnerabilities that we all carry with us as human beings, and that will have a direct effect on how an individual copes with the effects of their dementia. If a person has always placed great value on being in control of their lives and what happens around them, they are likely to struggle more with the consequences of dementia than someone who has always been happy to leave decisions to someone else. An extrovert may cope better with communal living than an introvert. Personality does not usually change as a result of having dementia. The ways in which people respond to stress and challenge are well-learnt behaviours. Talking to family members and friends about how people have coped with stress and adversity, and what has helped them through it, can offer clues about how they can best be assisted to cope with the challenges that living with dementia brings.

Social psychology (SP)

This is the social and psychological environment in which people with dementia find themselves. Primarily it is about the relationships between people. Kitwood's view of person-centred care for people with dementia was that it took place in the context of relationships. He wrote a great deal about this and the way in which social psychology could be supportive or damaging to people with dementia. As verbal abilities are lost, the importance of warm, accepting human contact through non-verbal channels becomes even more important than before.

With the onset of dementia, individuals are very vulnerable to their psychological defences being radically attacked and broken down. As the sense of self breaks down, it becomes increasingly important that it is held within the relationships that the person with dementia experiences. These relationships cannot be developed through the traditional therapy hour as in person-centred psychotherapy. Rather, the development of relationships occurs through the day-to-day interactions.

Writing in 2002, Christine Bryden suggested that Kitwood's Enriched Model could be utilised as a framework for counselling to help people living with dementia and their families to adapt to the challenges that dementia brings. People are diagnosed much earlier in the dementia trajectory so that they can engage directly with a more traditional counselling approach. Rehabilitative approaches are of necessity going to be individualised. Life story, personality and identity are central to approaches to help people make a good adjustment.

The individual experience of dementia will be determined in part by the social environment. Much can be done to ensure that the social environment is generally supportive of the needs of people with dementia. We return to this in greater depth in Chapter 6. When trying to determine an individualised plan of care, however, the way in which people respond to their surroundings and what triggers positive or negative reactions is important to assess at all stages.

Putting individualised care into practice

The indicators in the individual lives element of VIPS primarily need to be led by those setting the clinical or care standards within the care organisation. These indicators are about the processes that operate to ensure that care is delivered to a high standard.

As leaders for care standards within health and social care, sometimes it feels that all we can do is to keep the standards safe and prevent adverse events. Ensuring that health and safety and statutory legislation is met, keeping up with the latest developments and reporting on every activity imaginable mean that clinical leaders often feel overwhelmed by the level of demands upon them. If you are in a senior position in a care organisation, you will recognise this only too well.

Providing person-centred care that really takes individuals' lives seriously is a tough challenge. It is easy to skim the surface when it comes to the lives of people with dementia. The fact that you are reading this chapter means that you take this endeavour seriously and have a desire to dig deeper.

The questions that follow relate to these key areas. We outline why they are of importance to person-centred care and how you might think about changing the issues raised.

1. Care and support planning: Do our care and support plans promote individual identity showing that everyone is unique, with hopes, fears, strengths and needs?

Individualised assessment and analysis sets a basis from which interventions can be designed for enhancing well-being by appropriately matching activity and occupation to people living with dementia or reducing disturbed mood or behaviour. Many other interacting factors are likely to need consideration, such as level of dependency and a range of socio-economic, gender, ethnic or cultural differences.

Kitwood's Enriched Model of dementia, discussed earlier, is a good place to start in ensuring that a wide range of needs are covered. The person-centred care planning templates (May *et al.* 2009) provide an excellent basis for this. They identify 'Biography', 'Personality', 'Lifestyle', 'Life at the moment', 'Health and cognitive support needs' and 'Capacity for doing' as key domains.

In the Enriched Opportunities Programme (Brooker and Woolley 2007; Brooker *et al.* 2011), four different domains were addressed for each individual to help identify ways of optimising well-being.

The first domain was cognitive ability and engagement capacity. How does this person think? How do they communicate? How do they relate to the world? How do they relate to objects? This helps in planning the level that a person can engage with activities and what type of support they will need.

The second domain was life history. What experiences from the person's past could hold clues to improving and maintaining well-being now? This provides information as to what activities will be familiar and enjoyed. It also identifies objects that could trigger positive memories and actions. This involved the completion of life-story books and life boxes, either completed with the person or with the help of family members.

The third domain was personality. What is this person like? What motivates them? What influences their mood? This provides clues as to what the person enjoys and doesn't enjoy. This was completed through observations and by discussion with the key worker and family.

The final area was an assessment of current interests. What happens day to day that brings this person to life? What delights them? What creates a good day or a bad day for them? This provides the establishment of everyday opportunities that can bring real joy. This was completed through observations and by discussion with the key worker and family.

Organisational culture must help to ensure a focus on supporting individuals' lives, rather than creating lives for individuals that fit with the organisation. Do care and support plans focus on the physical tasks of care or do they attend to the whole person, and how they can be supported well each day? The origin of care plans can demonstrate a lot about an organisation and the support it provides. Why do they take the form they take? How are they used on a day-to-day basis? Who is involved in creating them?

Care planning processes that are designed and used in a certain way because of outside forces such as regulatory requirements or policies are not automatically going to lead to person-centred care experiences, however well intentioned. However, those designed to best capture and represent the person and best help support staff to focus on the person will encourage the norms of care on the ground: *we constantly look to make things better, we help people to enjoy places where they spend time* and *we help people to be active in a way that fulfils them every day*. This requires that *leadership protects front-line service delivery* in relation to factors such as regulation, organisational changes and policies to best encourage person-centred care. It is not that physical records are not important, but that their format and use need to be determined by what works and helps on the ground, rather than being an end in themselves.

In this first example, a care worker explains how different staff contribute on a daily basis to care planning for their residents:

The carers trial out care and work out what works for that individual and then we inform the nurses who then write it up in the care plans...at handover we discuss people's care. One lady does not like taking her medication. Her daughter-in-law is a GP. So what we have found to work is if we say to the resident, your daughter-in-law knows what medication you have been prescribed and approves of it and then the resident does take it. So we pass over that information in handover and it gets written into the notes... We wouldn't trial something with a resident without discussing it with the nurses...[they] may know more about why not to do something... So they provide a link between care on the floor, knowledge about each of the residents and the care plan writing.

However, in the next example a paper-focused approach to care planning (which the manager felt she could not avoid due to organisational and local authority demands) led to the following, frequent observation on the ground:

[As residents sit down to lunch] a carer asks second carer about daily dietary records for residents who haven't eaten yet. The other carer replies, 'Just record a spoonful.' This shows that care plans are a care task here rather than a product of the care given, to the extent that we record something even when it hasn't been done.

In this workplace, care staff were seen to be praised for completing their care records fully before finishing their shift.

Part 2 (page 190) provides questions to help you assess your organisation's performance on this indicator.

2. Regular reviews: Do we recognise and respond to change?

The needs of people with dementia change over time. We all have changing needs, but it is particularly important to be aware of this when working with people who may have progressive conditions. The pace of change will vary on an individual basis. For some the pace will be slow – so much so that it is easy to overlook subtle problems that may be causing a sense of failure in the person with dementia. For this reason, it is important that there is a fail-safe procedure so that everyone's care plan gets looked at every six months, at the least, to ensure that it is still meeting needs. On the other hand, there will be people whose needs change very quickly either because of the nature of their dementia or because of some other unstable physical health condition. Structures should be in place so that care plans can be reviewed quickly when necessary.

Building good relationships with local mental health teams or specialist services can help ensure that health and well-being is maintained at the optimal level. They can be useful where there are issues of significant deterioration, worsening confusion or depression.

An organisational culture that embraces change – one in which *we constantly look to make things better* – is absolutely crucial to achieving person-centred care on the ground to the extent that in a positive culture it is a norm of care, meaning that *not* to see it happening should be viewed as strange and prompt questions. However, change in these circumstances is purposeful and person-focused. It should come about because people change (often on an hourly basis), and therefore support needs to be able to change as well to accommodate this. Change that is driven by other needs, without considering the implications for people and those who provide their support, will lead to difficulties and less positive care experiences.

Embedding this sort of attitude and approach to change in an organisation or service requires that *front-line staff are empowered and supported* through management and leadership to create and sustain this change in their daily work. There is little point in expecting support staff to change and adapt to a person's well-being needs if the expectations on them and their work remain fixed. In these contradictory circumstances, support staff will face untenable conflicts between meeting people's needs and well-being and meeting the expectations of their leaders and organisations.

> Here, a head of care explains that reviewing care for residents needed to be a daily task, and one that everyone has a role in:
>
> > [Care and nursing staff] record any changes. So anyone, like I picked up straightaway. You know, rather than going and disturb [the] report, because…then you only hear one end don't you? I mean we've got 65 residents here. So I can immediately pick up anything, and if there's something, I might go then and talk to whoever's in charge to find out what's happening. You know, if someone's been poorly in the night or, you know…it's something that we bang on all the time… It's keeping care plans up to date… I have to audit the care plans anyway, so I make sure that they're being kept up to date as well, that they're accurate.

Part 2 (page 191) provides questions to help you assess your organisation's performance on this indicator.

3. Personal possessions: Do people have their favourite and important things around them? Do we know why they're meaningful for them?

As dementia progresses, people will obtain much greater comfort from wearing clothes that look familiar and using objects that are well known, rather than getting to grips with new possessions. The reasons for this are twofold. First, familiar items are a touchstone in a world that feels increasingly alien to people living with dementia. They link the present with the past, the unfamiliar with the known. Second, as dementia progresses, people often lose the ability to learn how to use new objects quickly, whereas with old objects the patterns are well learnt. Most of us have the experience of turning on a lamp with which we are familiar without even consciously thinking about where the switch is. With a new lamp we have to stop and think. It is the latter action that becomes difficult to manage in dementia. Surround the person with things that are familiar and they will be more at ease. When new things need to be purchased, try to buy the same make or model or buy clothes in the same material as ones that were cherished.

Regardless of how and where care and support are provided, personal possessions need to be considered in how support is set up and provided. For a residential care organisation this may be about how possessions, furniture and furnishings are introduced and used in a communal environment. For those providing care at home, it may be around making sure those items that are important are within reach or that equipment needed for care does not dominate the environment. In the hospital ward, this is about what personal items can be used to orient and comfort a person in such an alien and disorienting environment. In all of these situations using knowledge of the person and actively involving family and friends becomes central.

The role of personal possessions in creating positive care cultures is shown through the ways in which possessions are used and thought about, rather than simply their existence. Possessions primarily help facilitate the norms of care that exist in positive care cultures. If personal possessions are available to use and interact with and staff know their significance, then regardless of the setting in which support is being provided, possessions help to make sure that we *help people to enjoy places where they spend time.* A personal item is not sat on a shelf in the person's bedroom (a static use of the environment) but is used to help the person make sense of the world – if a soft toy provides comfort, it is with the person whenever they may need that comfort. Personal possessions are also evidenced in use when *we help people to be active in a way that fulfils them every day.* Again, this is not an isolated, static event such as a once-a-month memory-box activity, but is an ongoing, everyday occurrence. If people find it hard to initiate occupation for themselves, are personal possessions used to enable them to occupy themselves in ways that is meaningful? A person may no longer be able to knit a blanket, but their bag of wool could accompany them everywhere so they can engage with the world in a sensory way by winding and touching the wool. Using such personal possessions in an active and thoughtful way requires that *we empower and support front-line staff* to make decisions for the people they support, so that they can act on their interactions with people. It is also a way in which *we all work together* to create an environment that is personally meaningful for someone.

> In the following observation, the easy availability of someone's personal photos helped staff connect with a gentleman whose verbal communication was often hard to understand and who reacted physically to the support given by staff:
>
> > [Shows Fred a photo of his father-in-law.] Fred laughs out loud. Both care workers are bowled over by the reaction they get and show him others: 'That's my children there'; 'That's my girls.' The care worker invites me over and talks me through the photos. She is very interested and knowledgeable about Fred's life. And really wants to share it with him and me. Fred is remembering and recalling names, including two identical-looking dogs who he can tell apart. The care worker says to me several times, 'I can't believe his reaction.' She brings another care worker to see it… They discuss putting together a wall display for him. Fred seems so engaged and happy throughout this exchange it is like he is a different person. Later on the care worker comes into the room and puts a thumb up to Fred and he returns it, saying something. 'I love you,' the care worker says, 'I love you too,' says Fred. Fred reaches [his] hand out and the care worker reaches back and holds [his] hand.

> Part 2 (page 192) provides questions to help you assess your organisation's performance on this indicator.

4. Individual preferences: Are a person's likes, dislikes, preferences and choices listened to, known about and acted upon?

If familiar objects are important in dementia care, then familiar foods, drinks, music and routines are even more so. Familiarity with day-to-day experiences helps to establish security, trust and comfort. As anxiety decreases, so does the likelihood that a person will try to 'go home' in an attempt to find the familiar. Helping staff to recognise the importance of this is central to raising their empathy for the people they support.

There is an increasing recognition that trying to ensure there is familiarity in long-held routines and preferences is an important way of helping people feel at ease. Sometimes people will be able to tell us about these routines and preferences for themselves. Other times, they will not, which is when getting this information from family and friends can be useful. We also need to make sure that we are attuned to the non-verbal ways in which a person can express satisfaction or dissatisfaction about what is happening to them. Again, ensuring that direct care staff know about these routines and preferences and use them every day can be difficult but is vitally important. There is little point in having such information if it is locked away in a filing cabinet.

However, keeping to routines and well-known preferences does not necessarily mean that things have to be the same every day. People will be as willing to try something new as they always were – and perhaps more so in some cases. It is important for staff to observe body language and reactions to new situations, to know what it is that works in the here and now.

As well as everyday routines and preferences it is important to think more broadly. If any of us are feeling vulnerable, then familiar touchstones of our cultural identity, our spirituality or religion and food, drinks and music with which we are familiar are likely to have a calming effect. Vulnerability, anxiety and alienation are more likely to increase if those elements are missing. Because the person with dementia may lack the internal resources and reasoning to protect themselves against alienation, this can be much more damaging to their sense of self than it would be if they had intact cognitive abilities. This means that we need to be able to tap into such cultural parts of a person's identity. This means we must move beyond simple generalisations and assumptions to drill down towards what aspects of these are meaningful to each person.

As with personal possessions, individual preferences are significant in creating positive cultures when they are in use actively and continually with care and support. If individual preferences are known about, watched for and acted upon, this results in care and support that exhibits the norms of care: *we constantly look to make things better, we help people to enjoy places they spend time* and *we help people to be active in a way that fulfils them every day.* Change occurs frequently because staff are sensitive and responsive to the communication of a person in the moment, accepting that what brought joy yesterday may not work today. The environment is constantly adapted to the needs of a person to suit the routines and preferences that they need. A person is meaningfully occupied and engaged with the world because staff know what they like and dislike and how best to engage with them. Moreover, *empowered and supported front-line staff,* who *all work together to deliver the best care* are much more likely to achieve these norms on the ground and thus reinforce a positive care culture on a daily basis.

In this observation a worker shows how different people's preferences were sought and honoured when giving support to get ready for bed:

> Care workers say to each other, 'Who shall we do first?' They approach a resident in their room about whether they want to go to the bible reading (in the lounge). They then approach all four residents in the lounge: 'Do you want to go to bed?', 'Are you tired, do you want to go to bed?'"Do you want to watch some more?' she asks each of them and carefully listens to their answers. She respects their answers – none of them want to go. Care worker announces: 'No one wants to go to bed yet! We'll come back later.' The staff then go to various bedrooms to check if those residents want to go to bed, several don't.

Part 2 (page 193) provides questions to help you assess your organisation's performance on this indicator

5. Life history: Are a person's important relationships, significant life stories and key events known about and referenced in everyday activities?

As dementia progresses, it becomes more difficult to hold on to the stories of one's life and to be able to tell others of the defining moments that shaped our identity. One of the jobs of caring for someone with dementia is to learn these key stories and hold this narrative for them. This can be used to improve self-esteem and to maintain an identity in the face of increasing confusion. As the capacity for engagement becomes more difficult, objects that trigger good feelings become increasingly important.

In the Enriched Opportunities Programme we used 'life boxes' that contained cherished objects. This was more meaningful to many than life story books or even photo albums:

> The life boxes help don't they because they've all got something in their life box. So we've learned new stuff where they've got... And that's good if you're on a different House Group and residents you're not familiar with or...they are quite helpful. (Residential care worker)

Past experiences of vulnerability and trauma, particularly those that happened in childhood or teenage years can often be relived during dementia, particularly if current events or activities have emotional resonance with these past experiences. For example, if someone has a history of abuse, they may find help with personal care activities particularly traumatic.

Staff providing care and support need to know about and use this information in their daily interactions. Moreover, everyone involved with the person will need to recognise that collecting and using such stories is an ongoing process and one that requires sensitivity, trust and a supportive relationship (with both the person and their friends/family) to make it work. How many of us could capture the significant events of our lives in a four-page 'care plan' document, right at a time of great change and turmoil? Would anyone share life moments that brought great sadness or fear with just anybody? Do our 'next of kin' know everything about us? The answer to each of these questions is a resounding 'no'. Therefore, the way we approach life history for people we support must recognise and respond to the deeply personal, complex and ever-evolving nature of every individual's life story.

Again, positive care cultures show that it is the *use* of life history that helps create a person-centred experience for people rather than its existence alone. In cultures where *we all matter to each other*, people are known, know others and have opportunities to share and use such information within normal day-to-day interactions. As a visitor or a family member, if I feel connected to the care worker and feel that I know them and they value me, I am far more likely to share personally significant moments for my partner or parent, or in our relationship, because we interact based on trust and respect, and I know (from what I see) that the information will be put to good use. In particular, life histories were especially important to ensure that front-line staff were able to *help people to be active in a way that fulfils them every day*, precisely because they provide information about what might be meaningful and fulfilling for a person. Without thought and use of this information, attempts at engagement or occupation were routine and depersonalised. A cat is just a cat unless you know that someone has never lived without one, is afraid of them or is comforted by being helped to stroke one.

In this example a team leader explains what makes a good care worker for people living with dementia:

> You have to try and understand the residents, you know, try and get as much information as you can about their previous life before they came in here, you know, what they did, their family members, what they like, their hobbies before, you know, and try and speak to as many family members as you can, because you get a lot of information that way. Try and find out little things they like, you know, little sayings. I try and pick up on something that makes them smile, something that brings back happy memories.

This focus on life story and its application led to some wonderful observations of care and support on the ground in this care home:

> [The] care worker now comes and sits with Lola, Paul, Jo and some other residents in a circle. He says to Lola [in reply to her comment]: 'You're not sure you want me? Well, kick me out if you want.' He starts to chat to Lola about the periodic table (she was a chemistry teacher). Another staff member comes over to Jo and asks him where Lancashire is after a previous discussion when staff couldn't decide (Jo is good with geography). The care worker continues to chat with the group – uses prompts, residents' knowledge and contributions to keep it going – it continues for a good 40 minutes.

Part 2 (page 194) provides questions to help you assess your organisation's performance on this indicator.

6. Activity and occupation: Is a person's day full of purpose and engagement with the world, regardless of their needs and abilities?

Boredom and lack of meaningful activity is rife in care for older people generally, but particularly for those with more advanced dementia who often find it difficult to initiate or sustain activities and who may be outpaced by goal-oriented activities. Finding things that interest and sustain people can be a challenge. As well as knowing what is meaningful to each individual, understanding the capabilities of individuals with regard to their level or severity of dementia is likely to be important for providing suitable activities. In the early stages, adapting and maintaining existing interests in sports, gardening, pets, games, crafts and creative activities is productive. Creating life story resources and playlists of favourite music can also beneficial at this time and can be a great resource as dementia progresses. In the middle stages of dementia, switching to activities that require less cognitive load, such as creative activities including music, dancing and drama as well as physical activities such as walking, swimming and structured exercise, can be beneficial. In the later stages more sensory engagement such as aromatherapy, massage, creative art forms and sensory stimulation might be most appropriate for people with the highest levels of cognitive and functional impairment (Perrin, May and Milwain 2008).

Developing a firm evidence base of what works for whom, when and in what setting is a difficult task. Given the heterogeneity of this population, the varied skill level of staff and the enormous variety of settings where activities take place alongside the problems of finding suitable outcome measures, it is not surprising that the research evidence for many activity-based interventions can be difficult to be definitive about. Nonetheless, from a practice perspective, seeing someone light up with delight when engaged in an activity that has meaning for them is evidence enough that this is a worthwhile endeavour. It is applying occupation and activity as part of regular care practice that poses the real challenge.

How this can be achieved in all sorts of settings requires careful consideration. Who has responsibility for ensuring that service users have access to fun and meaningful occupation on a day-to-day basis? How is this provided? When does it happen – once a week or at every opportunity? How is it reviewed to ensure it meets the needs of individuals? Do we know how much time each of the people we support spends engaged or disengaged?

Activity organisers or coordinators are employed by some care providers to try to meet these needs for occupation. In the USA, Canada and Australia, the role of 'recreational therapist' has been developed. In the Enriched Opportunities Programme (Brooker *et al.* 2011) the specialist role of 'locksmith' was developed in order to meet this need in nursing homes and extra-care housing. In the Focussed Intervention Training and Support (FITS) into Practice Intervention (Brooker *et al.* 2015) the role of the Dementia Care Coach and the Dementia Practice Development Coach led on reducing anti-psychotic medication but also in providing meaningful activity for care home residents. Having someone take a lead on this aspect of care can greatly improve the chances that enjoyable and meaningful occupation will become a feature of everyday life. In any long-term service setting, however, there also has to be an appreciation that all staff from direct care workers through to management share in the responsibility for the provision of fun and occupation that give meaning and structure to life and stave off boredom.

'Activity' is not about having a predetermined schedule of events, or solely about bringing external events or activities in, and it is just as important for a person who is being supported to live at home or on a hospital ward as it is for someone in residential care. It is about finding and taking every opportunity to engage with a person or help them to engage with the world. It is easy for those with intact cognition and busy lives to underestimate drastically how much cognitive power and physical ability it takes to stave off boredom. When someone's ability to make sense of the world and what is going on around them is impaired, then occupying oneself, finding purpose and having an effect in the world becomes significantly harder to do. Good care for someone living with dementia requires supporters to recognise that they must now help a person with this, in exactly the same way that they may need to provide assistance to eat, to stay safe or to take care of personal hygiene.

The presence of meaningful engagement and occupation was so significant to a positive organisational culture that it was a norm of care in its own right: *we help people to be active in a way that fulfils them every day.* Crucially, positive care cultures existed where meaningful engagement and occupation were seen and acted on as being absolutely integral to good care, rather than as an added extra. This meant that everyone in the environment, particularly front-line care staff, needed to see it as part of their role, and so *empowerment and support for front-line staff* was crucial. If activities were viewed only as the domain of certain staff or something that only happened when spare time was available or when an event was happening then the culture did not result in positive care experiences.

Moreover, this feature also demonstrates the importance of thinking about people's individual lives as a whole (all of the VIPS indicators) rather than ticking a box related to 'activities'. It is only by knowing the individual well (whether through in-depth life histories or close knowledge of their communication and what it means in the here and now) that an activity, event, conversation, item or interaction becomes meaningful. Care or support without individualisation is functional at best. Good experiences of care and support are ones that are meaningful to the person – ones that add value to the moment by making it joyful or reducing its distress.

Here, a relative explained something she really appreciated about her mum's care home, something that made it stand out for her:

> Oh there's always something going on. I get dizzy sometimes! …I mean they're doing music and movement now, tomorrow will be knit and natter so you get a different group up there… We'll be having parties in the New Year put on by the Committee. There'll be loads going on over Christmas, for those who want it. Art class on a Monday. The one-to-ones as well, which I think are really important…they'll just have a sit and pamper, they'll have the manicure done or a little massage of their feet in the hot steam bath. Personal things like that. Or sometimes they'll be read to…it was 'let's play Scrabble'. So, all sorts of things like that really. Or just sat holding hands, which is sometimes what we all need don't we? I mean I've gone into the little lounge up here and I've seen a member of staff just sat there holding, and talking quietly to a resident, calming them and making them feel wanted and loved. So what more can we ask?

The activities coordinator at the same home explained that her approach was to encourage everyone to be involved in keeping people occupied:

> You know, it's just day to day really. [Care staff involvement] means everybody is getting some sort of stimulation…and there's a lot of good communication going on, you know. I think it's also [care staff] knowing, 'What can we do, we need this, what about it can we get it?' and all their ideas is just going with them really as best I can.

Part 2 (page 195) provides questions to help you assess your organisation's performance on this indicator.

Summary

Element 2 of person-centred care is about providing care on an individual basis where people are known about and accepted in their entirety – not just because of their diagnostic label. The degree to which organisations support individuals' lives can be seen in many organisational processes around assessment and care planning. It is also evident in how people lead their day-to-day lives and whether this is based around their lifestyles, preferences and needs for activity and occupation.

5

Personal Perspectives

Element 3 of person-centred care is looking at the world from the perspective of the person living with dementia

Looking at the world from the perspective of the person with dementia: recognising that each person's experience has its own psychological validity, that people act from this perspective and that empathy with this perspective has its own therapeutic potential.

Key indicators for care providers of taking the perspective of the person living with dementia

- **Communication is key**: Are we alert to all the ways that people living with dementia communicate and are we skilled at responding appropriately?

- **Empathy and acceptable risk**: Do we put ourselves in the position of the person we're supporting and think about the world from their point of view?

- **Physical environment**: Is this a place that helps someone living with dementia to feel comfortable, safe and at ease?

- **Physical health**: Are we alert to, responsive to and optimising people's health and well-being?

- **Challenging behaviour as communication**: Do we always consider and act on what a person is trying to tell us though their behavioural communication? Do we look for underlying reasons rather than seeking to 'manage' it?

- **Advocacy**: Do we speak out on behalf of people living with dementia to make sure their rights, respect and dignity are upheld?

In person-centred care it is the subjective experience of the individual that is important. Even when a person's subjective experience may differ from what others see as 'reality', it is the person's perspective rather than ours (or anyone else's) that needs to be paramount. This is because the fundamental starting point for helping someone is trying to understand the world as they see it. Therapeutic approaches that follow a person-centred approach (such as Rogers 1961) see entering the frame of reference of the individual and understanding the world from their point of view as key to working successfully and supportively with someone. Part of taking the perspective of the person with dementia as a starting point for care is the ability to relate to them directly, seeing them as a fellow human being.

Kitwood recognised the centrality of understanding the individual needs of people with dementia to give a focus for interventions. He asserts very strongly that without empathy the care environment would remain cold (1997b). Stokes (2000) also highlights the understanding of subjective experience as key to working in a person-centred way with so-called challenging behaviour. Clare *et al.* (2003) define person-centred approaches to dementia care as focusing on individual experiences: 'understanding the experience of dementia in terms of the person's psychological responses and social context, and aiming to tailor help and support to match individual needs' (Clare *et al.* 2003, p.251).

One of the most evident changes in the dementia care field since the first edition of this book has been the richness and power of the voices of people living with dementia speaking out in their own right. Up until relatively recently, it was thought that, because of the symptoms of disorientation and dysphasia, people experiencing dementia could not communicate anything in a meaningful or reliable fashion. Indeed, this is still the prevailing opinion in some countries and cultures. Over recent years there has been a shift in focus. This is, in part, to do with the person-centred care movement itself. As people with dementia have stepped out from behind the disease label, the recognition that they have something important to say has grown. There is also a much greater acknowledgement that speaking directly on one's own behalf is deeply empowering. Also, people with dementia are being diagnosed generally at an earlier stage. Alzheimer's Societies and Associations worldwide now have the representation of people living with dementia as a core part of their mission. 'Nothing about us, without us' has been a slogan of the disability rights movement for many years and has now finally been accepted as being true in dementia too (Bryden 2015). Personal accounts of living with dementia are very powerful and have been instrumental in the development of policy initiatives at the national and international level. People with dementia are seen as the real experts by experience.

In dementia research, phenomenological research into the early experience of Alzheimer's (Clare 2002; Sabat 2001) is now well established. In quality-of-life research, self-report measures on subjective well-being (Brod *et al.* 1999) and quality of life are now available (Smith *et al.* 2005). There is now a body of evidence that people with dementia can answer interview questions in a reliable manner and can be involved directly in the research process. In dementia care practice, engaging directly with people with dementia in a therapeutic sense has been established in the literature for some time (Cheston, Jones and Gillard 2003) although therapeutic practice of providing counselling services for people living with dementia is not widespread. Post-diagnostic support interventions recognise that helping people come to terms directly with what is happening to them is important for long-term adjustment (Dröes *et al.* 2003).

How can we appreciate the perspective of someone with dementia at more advanced stages?

The inclusion of the direct accounts from people living with dementia has been a very important strength of the development of a more inclusive person-centred approach. It is important to remain aware, however, that the experience of a person with advanced dementia or with additional physical or sensory disabilities will be very different to someone in earlier stages or someone who is relatively fit and healthy in other respects.

Putting oneself in the shoes of someone living with advanced dementia is not an easy or trivial process. Can any of us really know what it is like to be another person? The answer is no. Treating someone 'as I would like to be treated' is not the same as genuinely seeing the world through another's eyes. Therefore, we need constantly to attempt to be reflective and persistent in our efforts to see the world from a different perspective, precisely because it is a hard thing to do. In addition to listening to direct accounts, Kitwood (1997c) described various ways by which dementia care practitioners could deepen their empathy toward people with dementia. These can be used in professional development, training and in day-to-day reflective practice.

They include:

- attending carefully to the actions and words of people with dementia

- using imagination to understand the experience of dementia.

Attending carefully

As verbal communication becomes more difficult, paying close attention to a person's non-verbal behaviour or piecing together fragmented speech becomes increasingly important. The work of John Killick and Kate Allan (2001) has been extremely influential in helping practitioners attend to the person with dementia in imaginative, creative and reflective ways. Killick and Allan (2006) describe their work with people with advanced dementia who are near to death, based on 'coma work' principles and using video and sound recordings, paying very close attention to detail.

> Here, a care worker from a care home that participated in the CHOICE project explains how she communicates with people who have limited verbal communication as a result of their dementia:
>
> So often if I sit there and like a lady taps the table and I tap it back, and sometimes she'll sit up. Or one lady, she calls out in like 'Oh my daddy,' and you say 'Oh my daddy,' and she'll look up at you. Whereas if you just be like 'Oh Mary,' or just carry on talking about something else, you know, you won't always respond. So if you kind of use the same communication she's using it's quite interesting what reaction you get. (Care worker)

Another way of helping people to attend more carefully is through using a structured observation technique. Kitwood and colleagues developed Dementia Care Mapping (DCM) as a means of helping care practitioners to heighten their awareness of the needs of people with dementia in long-term care and to appreciate their experience of life. Kitwood defined DCM thus: 'DCM is a serious attempt to take the standpoint of the person with dementia, using a combination of empathy and observational skill' (Kitwood 1997a, p.4). The spread of DCM worldwide has been remarkable. The DCM tool and training materials have been translated into ten different languages, and it is estimated that up to 12,000 practitioners have been trained in DCM since the early 1990s (Brooker and Surr 2015). Many practitioners who have used DCM attest to the powerful personal impact of observing in this way. Vera Bidder, a nursing assistant working on a hospital project described by Tracy Packer (Packer 1996), described how DCM changed her empathic response to people with dementia in her care:

> Shortly after the [DCM] course I became very conscious of the detractions that were still going on... I was bathing a person who was having difficulty forming a conversation. The door was flung open and the curtain pulled back. I protested, and the response was 'It's only a patient!' I was livid because it felt like it was me. I was the person having their privacy invaded. I found myself apologising to the person involved even though it wasn't my fault. (p.22)

Using the imagination

Using the imagination to put oneself in the place of someone trying to cope with the symptoms of dementia is a very powerful means of increasing empathy. The symptoms of disorientation, dysphasias and dyspraxias are often described, but it is how these make people feel that is often overlooked.

Working in the field of dementia care, you learn very quickly that the emotional reactions that people with dementia experience are as strong as they ever were. Although there is a decline in cognitive abilities, there is no decline in depth of feeling. Indeed, for many people, emotions appear stronger than ever, partly because of the decline in the volitional control of emotions that can be part and parcel of dementia. Anger, joy, grief and excitement are often easily accessed. Front-line staff need to tap into the emotion first and respond accordingly. Thinking carefully about how we talk about and communicate people's emotions in the course of care and support can drastically change the extent to which a person's own perspective is highlighted or hidden from view. Compare the following daily recordings about Mrs Jones and think about whose perspective is captured:

- 'Mrs Jones became difficult and aggressive during personal care.'

- 'When I was helping Mrs Jones to go to the toilet she screamed and tried to push me away with her hand as I pulled her underwear down.'

Both these sentences describe the same event, but in the first it is the recorder's interpretation that is written down and therefore passed on to whoever reads the record. However, in the second, we gain a (small) insight into Mrs Jones's feelings and experience and this is more likely to prompt us to reflect on what we are doing and how: if we get a sense that Mrs Jones is frightened and feels violated we are far more likely to change what we are doing to help her feel safe.

As dementia progresses there is often a constant interplay between memories that are well stored and what is going on in the here and now. Past events and memories feel much more present than recent ones. Present events will trigger past memories. What is happening in the present moment has a significant impact on how the person feels. We can all tap into our own experiences of feeling lost, alone and scared, or safe, comforted and like we belong, and these can be used to help us imagine what someone may feel like if they only have these past experiences to draw on and if their moment-to-moment experiences are negative.

> In this short exchange observation here, a care worker shows how empathy and acknowledgement of her own feelings helped her to reach out and comfort someone in need:
>
> A resident is sat at the table calling out: 'I'm so alone, alone. My mum and dad are gone.' A care worker picks up her cup of tea and takes a seat next to him, saying: 'My mum and dad are gone too, so shall we be alone together?'

Encouraging staff to tap into this natural resource helps to decrease the distance between 'us' and 'them' and recognise that we are all human and dependent on each other for well-being. It helps us all to recognise that we can make a huge difference to people's experiences in the moment and, crucially, that when impaired cognition makes it hard to orient yourself in the present, imagine the future or recall the recent past, it is the *moment* that matters most of all. Dementia may well affect my ability to remember that someone came to help me to the toilet last time I asked. It also makes it very hard for me to make sense of the strange environment of the hospital ward and reassure myself that I am safe and looked after. This means that how you make me feel right *now* is the most important thing, and that feeling will be what I carry forward into the rest of my day.

Role play and other methods that engage poetic imagination are sometimes routes to epiphanic knowledge (Hawkins 2005) – so-called 'light-bulb moments'. Film, poetry, fiction, personal accounts and observations, or conversations with clients, can all be a route to epiphanic knowledge. Novels and films that use the experience of someone living with dementia make this experience easier for people to access than it used to be, meaning that this becomes a more central part of our shared understanding of humanity.

Personal perspectives in practice

The indicators in the personal perspectives element of VIPS primarily need to be led by those who are responsible for the day-to-day management of front-line staff and the direct service environment. These indicators are about the way in which direct care staff respond to their caring role and how they demonstrate empathy with those they care for. However, it is important to remember that what front-line staff demonstrate on the ground is facilitated or restrained by the organisational culture in which they operate. So, if an indicator is not being achieved, we need to consider the solution and actions to take holistically, rather than simply demand staff 'do it better'.

Having responsibility for the operational management of a direct service team or leading shifts within a service is a tough job. It often feels as if everyone comes to you with their problems. Balancing the needs of an overworked staff group, covering shifts, dealing with sickness, new service users, deaths and illness, worried or angry relatives and having to attend meetings that go on for hours are all in a day's work for people in this position. All this can easily take precedence over being a role model for staff and ensuring that their day-to-day interactions are of a high standard and they receive the support they need. If no one is complaining, then it is easy to think that there is no problem.

Providing person-centred care that really takes the perspective of people with dementia – particularly those with more advanced dementia – is a tough challenge. The fact that you are reading this chapter means that you take this endeavour seriously and have a desire to be proactive in ensuring that the people you support get the best possible opportunity to have their needs understood.

What follows is a series of questions to help care providers benchmark where they are in terms of the personal perspective element of person-centred care. These questions will help you explore how well your service and staff try to look at life from the perspective of the person with dementia. They will also prompt you to think about what might need to change and how each indicator is linked to the organisational culture of the service.

1. Communication is key: Are we alert to all the ways that people living with dementia communicate and are we skilled at responding appropriately?

In order to know a person's opinion, it is important that they are asked directly! However, it is surprising how often this basic courtesy and social interaction does not occur in services for people with dementia. This happens for a number of reasons. The first is the belief that the person with dementia cannot make a reliable comment, and the second is that it will take too long. Although people may lose the capacity to make truly informed choices about abstract decisions as time goes by, the evidence is that people can make reliable decisions about long-held preferences well into their dementia. Even if the capacity for understanding language is severely impaired, the non-verbal behaviour that accompanies being asked for permission or an opinion will not go unnoticed and will do much to convey to the person with dementia that they are worth bothering about.

Moreover, truly attentive staff will take note of people's communication during and after an event or action has taken place and use it to build a picture of what works and does not work for this person. If someone struggles to answer a direct question or express an opinion easily, front-line staff may have to adopt a 'trial-and-error' approach to allow a person to experience the decision first-hand and then communicate their opinion. If the question 'Do you want to listen to some music today?' is too hard for a person to understand and decide upon in the abstract, truly attentive staff will support the person to listen to the music and then pay close attention to the person's non-verbal communication as to whether it is something that is enhancing to their well-being.

This is different from user involvement activities where people may be interviewed or surveyed about their views. What we are describing here is the everyday practice of asking for people's opinions on what they want to eat or drink, where they would like to sit and what they need to feel comfortable. On a day-to-day basis, are attempts made to discuss these sorts of issues directly with the person with dementia? Are the direct care staff good communicators generally? Do they recognise the barriers to communication due to cognitive disabilities and have strategies to overcome these?

When decisions need to be made that are either too complex or too abstract for the person living with dementia to make an informed decision about, do staff talk to people who know them well, who can often offer insight into their past preferences? Is this backed up by observations of the person in different situations to attempt or confirm a best estimation of their wishes?

The feature of organisational culture that helps or hinders good communication skills was *empowering and supporting front-line staff.* This is because, in order to employ good communication and, crucially, to respond to it, staff need to be able to act on what was communicated. If staff lack either the sense of responsibility or freedom to do this effectively, then communication, however skilled, feels futile because it cannot affect what happens next. As a front-line worker, in order to use my communication skills I need to know that I can act on what the person expresses to me. If I know that a person's choices and options are restricted (by expectations of others, rules governing what I can or cannot do or amount of tasks I have to complete) why and how would I see communication that truly allows expression from a person as being worthwhile? Asking someone what they would like to do, might yield the answer 'sit in sunshine'. If I know through experience that this is not permitted, or ever possible because of my other tasks, it is completely understandable that I might avoid, both consciously and unconsciously, asking the question or hearing the answer.

Each of the three norms of care, in which *staff constantly look to make things better, help people to enjoy places where they spend time* and *help people to be active in a way that fulfils them every day* all require good communication skills, because these actions happen in response to people's expressions, choices and opinions being acted on by staff. When people's voices are not heard or encouraged then decisions made from day to day are responsive only to organisational and staff demands.

In this example, a staff member shows attentive communication with a resident who was unable to speak more than singular words, and often could not find the right one, causing her frustration:

> The care worker is helping Ruby with her lunch. She says to Ruby, 'Is there something you don't like in there?'
>
> 'Yes.' A back and forth of short questions establishes that it's the runner beans.
>
> 'Okay, then we won't have any of them!' There is more exchange about whether she likes it or not. The care worker is very attentive to Ruby's facial expression. A little later the care worker says, 'Shall we give this dinner a miss?' Ruby replies, 'Yes!'
>
> 'Pudding?'
>
> 'Yes.'
>
> 'Rice pudding or a cake?'
>
> 'Yes.'
>
> 'Rice pudding *and* a cake?!'
>
> 'Yes'
>
> 'Okay, we'll try them all!'

Part 2 (page 197) provides questions to help you assess your organisation's performance on this indicator.

2. Empathy and acceptable risk: Do we put ourselves in the position of the person we're supporting and think about the world from their point of view?

There will be occasions when and decisions in which the person with more advanced dementia is unable to participate fully and put forward their own point of view. It is even more important then that staff are able to try to think things through from the viewpoint of the person with dementia. These sorts of issues are particularly important around issues of risk and considerations of safety. There can be tremendous pressure to err on the side of caution with regards to risk and to prioritise physical safety above all else. However, people with dementia are in danger of being kept so safe that they have no quality of life at all. Because of memory problems and impaired communication abilities, people with dementia often cannot express their wishes, and it is easier to prioritise safety so much that life becomes little more than keeping the body alive.

An empathic approach requires that we consider day-to-day activities and decisions in a way that balances their potentially positive impact on a person's emotional and physical well-being with any potential risks. All of us take risks every day; they are a fundamental part of life and human interaction with the world. A life without risks is one that is sterile and meaningless. Not being able to calculate risks for themselves should not mean that people with dementia are condemned to such a life. A good approach to risk is one that is empowering and seeks to reduce restriction (of all kinds) as much as possible, because freedom and control over our own actions are things that enhance all of our well-being.

However, all too often we still encounter stories of people's lives being stripped of all opportunity and excitement on the rationale of 'safety'. Empathy for a person's perspective requires us to acknowledge that 'safety' is a highly subjective concept that should not be seen only in narrow, physical terms. I may be physically safe from the 'risk' of falling over if I am kept sitting down in a chair all day, but do I *feel* safe? Is my emotional well-being being safeguarded by this approach? No, it is not. Not to mention the additional physical risks that are often inadvertently encouraged by such a 'risk-averse' attitude. If a person feels trapped and unsafe, they will understandably try to escape that feeling, often resorting to extreme actions to do so.

Considering only the physical aspects of safety neglects the fact that well-being requires more than this. Well-being is supported by experiences that bring support for psychological needs as well as physical ones. These are likely to include activities that carry an element of risk, such as walking in open air, carrying on hobbies despite physical frailties and trying new things. Good, person-centred support weighs the risks of an action against the *benefits* that it holds for the person's well-being and focuses on enabling a risk to happen as safely as possible rather than preventing the activity completely.

However, many of those working in settings to support people living with dementia continue to experience pressures to focus on risk prevention rather than risk enablement.

In the UK, legislation and guidance exist that encourage a risk-enablement approach, embedded in the perspective of the person themselves. The Mental Capacity Act 2005 (TSO 2005) and Department of Health guidance *Nothing Ventured, Nothing Gained* (2010) provide a positive framework for working in this empowering way. However, despite this, risk aversion is still very much evidenced in practice. This illustrates how strong the organisational and societal push towards risk aversion is. It takes consistent effort, strong will and great skill and knowledge to counter this cultural pressure.

There are hidden dangers and risks that threaten emotional well-being in the form of boredom, helplessness, depression and giving up. Often, it will be up to the person's support worker or a professional to advocate on behalf of their emotional well-being. Being able to use information about what the person enjoys doing now, how this relates to past wishes and being able to understand communication of well-being or ill-being is of essential importance. In order to put this into practice, are staff able to tell if a person with dementia is in a state of relative well-being or ill-being? Can they identify, describe and respond appropriately to verbal and non-verbal signs of well-being and ill-being? Is this done as part of a decision-making process about risk? Are staff supported to understand and apply any legislation concerning this area into their practice? Are these principles and issues around well-being and risk communicated clearly to friends and family who may understandably be concerned?

An organisational culture needs to ensure that staff are *empowered and supported* to act on the empathy they have for a person in order to give it life, just as they need to with a person's communication. In addition, particularly when thinking about risk, ability of *leadership to protect front-line service delivery* is absolutely crucial. A manager needs to be able to ensure that considerations of regulation, policy compliance, safety concerns etc. do not have a detrimental impact upon the freedom and well-being of people receiving support. These external factors are important and often designed to prevent poor-quality care or unacceptable risks to vulnerable people, but if simply passed to front-line staff, they will result in risk aversion, excessive paperwork and a focus on appearance of safety rather than evidence of safety through maximum well-being. A manager needs to support staff in working through these complex, ever-changing issues, allow learning (rather than punishment) from mistakes and near misses and be supported themselves by these outside factors to manage these complexities. Cultures in which *we all work together to deliver the best care* is also important in helping everyone to make decisions and work through these complex issues. This is because if we all have a practical understanding of a person's well-being and how it might be achieved then we are more focused on making something positive happen, rather than simply preventing negative events.

In this care home, we frequently saw pictures and heard talk of a recent trip to the seaside, which had been enjoyed by some of the residents living with dementia. The team leader explained how she had gone about arranging the trip and how the support of her manager was essential to making it possible, despite the many and varied risk assessments that needed to take place. The manager had described her organisation's approach to risk as one of, 'You need a reason *not* to do it, not a reason to do it.' The team leader explained:

> The trip originated from a conversation with Jo [resident] about where he would like to go if he could do anything he wanted. He said that he would choose to go back to Blackpool where he used to holiday as a boy. This sparked an idea and [I] decided they should do a day trip. I initially suggested it to staff and there was lots of negativity, they wanted to go somewhere closer. If I'd have listened to them then we'd have gone closer, just because you've got dementia, why does it mean you can only go up the street? [I] spoke to [activities coordinator] who thought it was fantastic and was very enthusiastic about it and [I] spoke to [manager] who said, 'We're doing it!'…we didn't want to pick those [residents] with whom it would be 'easy'. It was about those who would benefit. [I] volunteered to go, and other staff followed. Sometimes you've got to drive things through.

Part 2 (page 198) provides questions to help you assess your organisation's performance on this indicator.

3. Physical environment: Is this a place that helps someone living with dementia feel comfortable, safe and at ease?

People with more advanced dementia are often at the mercy of other people controlling their physical environment. Imagine being in your 80s, living with a dementia, being confined to a chair because you can no longer walk and sitting for ten hours a day in the same lounge in the same chair in the same position. The radio in the next lounge is constantly tuned to pop music you don't recognise; the TV in your lounge alternates between soap operas and children's programmes set at a constantly high volume; you cannot see out of any of the windows because the sills are above your eyeline; a loud call bell goes off at unpredictable intervals; a different bell goes off every time someone leaves or enters the front door; footsteps echo down the uncarpeted corridors; the hearing aid of the person sitting next to you whistles all day; and you are cold. This is the reality of the lived experience of many people living in care homes. Attention may have been paid to the physical design of such facilities – they may even have won architectural awards – but, unless the microenvironment is managed so that people are comfortable then such endeavour is worthless.

On a day-to-day basis, it is important that staff use their empathic skills to be actively aware of the comfort needs of people with dementia. Often, people with dementia may not be able to tell staff directly that they are in discomfort or they may not be able to work out for themselves how to alleviate discomfort. This may occur many times over the course of a day and night.

Let's consider a few such incidents that might occur in the morning. At breakfast, a cup placed too far away may get ignored and the person will not drink and remain thirsty; while getting dressed, a garment may be put on incorrectly causing skin to become sore; sitting in a chair by the window in the sun may cause the person to become too hot, and the glare of the sun into the room may mean they do not see the drink placed on the table next to them. The thirst continues. The person becomes anxious and begins to pace about, trying to find a way to stop the discomfort. None of these incidents on its own would trigger a major incident, but if allowed to continue, their cumulative effect could be devastating, leading to 'challenging behaviour' and very quick physical decline.

Incidents such as these can be picked up by everyone in the environment understanding the needs of people living with dementia and knowing that their observation skills and ability to respond are crucial – perhaps the difference between pain and comfort, happiness and anxiety or even life and death. In busy environments, it is easy for this sort of scenario to unfold unless steps are taken to minimise the risk of it happening.

Moreover, an awareness of the microenvironment from the perspective of the person is vitally important. Is consideration given to what the noise levels, light, smells and temperatures feel like to the person themselves, rather than busy staff dashing about? Observations or consciously putting oneself in the shoes of the person with dementia are, again, the only ways to ensure this is thought about and remedied.

Positive care cultures emphasised the importance of this, because constantly reflecting and *helping people to enjoy places where they spend time* is a norm of care. It meant that staff constantly thought about the issues in this indicator and took action to change them for the benefit of people. This is why the norms of care are so connected, because in order to respond to the environment there also needs to be norms of *constantly looking to make things better* and *helping people to be active in a way that fulfils them every day.*

For organisational culture, it is also important to think beyond the actions of front-line staff and consider the impact of organisational decision-making on the flexibility available within the environment. Do corporate decisions such as standardised colour schemes or installation of equipment etc. take into consideration the impact they have on people with dementia or consult with staff about how they may impact their ability to adapt to people's needs on a daily basis? A uniform approach to painting and decoration may look good in a brochure, but what if Mr Jones cannot recognise where his bedroom is? This also means that there is a need for *leadership to protect front-line service delivery* by acting as an intermediary between these decisions and the staff on the front line.

In these two contrasting examples, the extent to which staff and an organisation are able to use the environment for residents is highlighted. First, a care worker spoke about the changes she had recently made to the environment of her care home and the benefits it had:

> When I first worked downstairs there was nothing on the sides, there was nothing left out. We put the kettle away after every cup of tea that we made, we put the toaster away, all the locks was [on] the doors. There was nothing, there was no shelves, rummage [items], there was nothing at all around, [but now] the messier the better. And it's nice…when they rummage around through stuff. But then you find out more things about them as well. Like Britta, give her a pack of cards and she can do patience, can't she?

However, in a different care home this observation showed that even when good ideas were in place, how they were used was what mattered:

> Bedrooms have memory boxes outside. Betty's is covered in smudged finger marks, (I have seen her touch it a lot). There is a poem inside that talks about how much Betty likes to see her name; it says she will point and smile when she sees it. When I turn to Betty's bedroom door I see that it does not have her name on it.

Part 2 (page 199) provides questions to help you assess your organisation's performance on this indicator.

4. Physical health: Are we alert to, responsive to and optimising people's health and well-being?

As we saw in Chapter 4, people with dementia are prone to having physical health problems that can go undetected for long periods if staff around them are not vigilant about investigating causes of any sudden increase in confusion. When caring for a person with dementia, any sudden increase in the level of confusion should be treated with the suspicion that there could be a physical health problem contributing to the change. Physical fitness and comfort need to be taken seriously. Poor physical health greatly intensifies the impairments caused by dementia. Pain is often undetected in people with dementia, and the manifestations of the person's discomfort may be misperceived as 'challenging behaviour'. As people with dementia may have difficulty remembering episodes of pain or finding the words to describe their symptoms, the onus has to be on those providing direct care to be proactive in this respect.

Unaddressed sensory impairments such as not having the correct spectacles or functioning hearing aids often lie at the root of communication problems. If someone has poor visual perception and dysphasia due to their dementia, this only gets worse if they do not have all the help they can get from spectacles and hearing aids. Again, because of their dementia, an individual may not be able to say that they have lost their glasses or complain that their hearing aid no longer functions. Professionals and care staff have to be vigilant on their behalf.

Two features of positive care cultures are needed to help facilitate attentiveness to health and well-being. First, we need to *empower and support front-line staff* to act on their concerns, and this requires that they have the skills, know the boundaries of their roles within their own particular service and trust that their concerns (expressed on behalf of a person with dementia) will be acted upon by those who can administer or prompt medical interventions. Second, and of particular importance to services that do not have in-house access to primary or secondary health services (residential care homes, day care, care at home etc.), this will require the management of that service to be able to communicate appropriately and negotiate with external health services such as GPs, ambulance staff etc., and help their staff to do so as well. This is an aspect of *protecting front-line service delivery* and is, of course, a two-way process. Those external health services must also recognise and maximise their own role. We continue to hear of persistent difficulties in engaging appropriate healthcare support for people living with dementia. The time and energy that front-line staff often have to devote to such advocacy is time and energy that needs to be taken from elsewhere and thus will impact on people living with dementia.

A care worker in this home explains how communication between staff on a daily basis is essential to keep on top of physical health and well-being for their residents:

> That is very important. If a nurse passes over a piece of information such as a resident not taking their medication [without communication], I won't have a chance to say, 'Have you tried this or that approach with that person?' And they don't have the opportunity to say, 'I did try that approach and it didn't work,' then we can discuss this further. A solution can come up when you do that, when you have those type[s] of communication. You see if a resident has had their medication stopped the nurse can tell you what to look for, what effects of stopping that medication may be. How can you support your residents if you do not have that information and you cannot feed back what effects may be happening for a resident? Writing someone has had an unsettled night isn't enough information to provide the care the resident needs. You need to know more, the context, was the person up and down out of bed, going to the toilet frequently, drinking, or calling for their mum. We need to think about why they were unsettled and what we can do to help them today.

Part 2 (page 200) provides questions to help you assess your organisation's performance on this indicator.

5. Challenging behaviour as communication: Do we always consider and act on what a person is trying to tell us though their behavioural communication? Do we look for underlying reasons rather than seek to 'manage' it?

A great deal has been written about the need to understand so-called 'challenging behaviour' from the perspective of the person with dementia (Power 2014). These behaviours are sometimes referred to as behavioural and psychological symptoms of dementia (BPSD). This is an umbrella term for the secondary symptoms of dementia such as agitation, wandering, hallucinations, delusions, depression, anxiety, aggression and shouting out, which can be very common in dementia. These are the types of behaviour listed on the Neuropsychiatric Inventory (NPI) and are sometimes also called neuropsychiatric symptoms, challenging behaviours or distress behaviours. These are the problems that often lead to people being prescribed anti-psychotic medication or being physically restrained or sedated.

In person-centred care, we try to see meaning in all behaviour and use this as a starting point for trying to help. The first step is in trying to understand the function of the behaviour for the individual and what the person is trying to tell us by the behaviour. This is particularly evident when people with dementia are in distress but cannot explain this through normal channels. Thus we might see the person act in a way that has been labelled as challenging, with behaviours such as verbal or physical aggression, self-harm, shouting out, repetitive questioning, escape behaviours, paranoid behaviours, accusatory behaviours, socially inappropriate behaviours and sexually inappropriate behaviours. These are very distressing events both to the person experiencing them and to those in a caring role.

A person-centred response would be to see the challenge as one for us as caregivers, not the person themselves. The event or behaviour challenges us, as a team, to find out the reasons underlying the behaviour and to help the person achieve a state of well-being, based on the understanding that if we achieve that well-being, then the 'need' being communicated though the behaviour has been met. In understanding the perspective of the person living with dementia and using this as part of our detailed analysis, we can then have a plan that supports personhood and thus is likely to reduce most of the behaviours that are challenging to respond to.

The terms themselves are contentious. In our general work with care teams we usually use the term 'distress' or 'distress behaviours' to indicate the reactive nature of what is often occurring. As Victor Frankl (2004) said, 'An abnormal reaction to an abnormal situation is normal behaviour' (p.32). Distress is often interpreted as being part of the dementia itself. However, the majority of BPSDs are the result of untreated delirium, untreated pain, lack of understanding of cognitive capacity, poor nutrition and hydration, poor communication, lack of knowledge about the person's history, poor general care, boredom and unmet emotional needs. In addition, many of these problems occur through lack of understanding of what it is like to be a person living with dementia. This understanding does not happen automatically. There is often a gap in the experience between those living with dementia and those providing care and support. This gap widens as the dementia progresses.

This is the arena in which skilled care really counts and really makes a difference. By seeking to understand why the distress is occurring and by providing supportive interactions where people are met with warmth, inclusion, respect and empathy, people will feel less confused and more relaxed, socially confident and joyful. Al Power in the USA provides many examples from a strengths-based approach to illustrate this many times over (Power 2014). This will directly reverse or decrease those feelings underpinning the occurrence of BPSD. This does not mean that the dementia has gone away *but* it does mean that the person feels less as if they are losing their mind.

As Christine Bryden writes:

> The world goes much faster than we do, whizzing around, and we are being asked to do things, or to respond, or to play a game, or to participate in group activities. It is too fast, we want to say 'Go away, slow down, leave me alone, just go away' and maybe we might then be difficult, not co-operative. Challenging behaviour? I believe that this is 'adaptive behaviour', where I am adapting to my care environment. (Bryden 2005, p.128)

The reasons underlying distress can usually be understood by reference to the Enriched Model of dementia. Is there something about this person's cognitive disability that means they are misinterpreting or becoming overwhelmed by their situation? Is there something in their past life that is being triggered by their current situation that is causing distress? Is there a mismatch between their preferences and needs and what the current environment is offering? Is there an untreated physical complaint that is causing an increase in confusion or pain? Is the social interaction and engagement meeting their personhood needs?

The practice of being proactive, and always considering what a situation may look and feel like to the person with dementia, should lead to a lower incidence of distress. We have worked on many specialist facilities that are characterised by an atmosphere of relative calm. To the casual visitor, it will look as if staff are doing very little apart from spending time with people as needed. This belies the fact that the team will have spent time learning all about the viewpoints of those for whom they are caring and putting it into everyday practice. The distress reoccurs very quickly if people are placed back in situations where staff do not have the ability to try to put themselves in the position of the person for whom they are caring.

There is a strong track record in clinical psychology for using a functional or behavioural analysis approach to understand why people are experiencing the sorts of problems described as challenging. Functional, analysis-based interventions are sometimes called the ABC approach because they begin with a very clear description of the target behaviour (B); the events that lead up to it (A – the antecedents) and what happens as a result (C – the consequences). Functional analysis takes behavioural analysis to a much more sophisticated level in recognising that the relationship between antecedents, behaviours and consequences is often non-linear and complex (James 2011).

Positive care cultures will enable this thoughtful, reflective and responsible approach to behavioural communication to occur. In particular, *empowered and supported front-line staff* will be able to take responsibility and make decisions to prevent and adapt in response to distress behaviours and they will be able to reflect constantly on the well-being needs of that person and how they are being met or not met. It is important to recognise the day-to-day support that staff themselves might need in thinking about and responding to challenges such as this.

Responding reflectively and patiently to someone who may be causing physical or emotional hurt or doing something that makes your (already stressful) job appear much harder is much easier said than done. Staff need practical and emotional support for their *own* personhood needs to ensure they have the resources to dig deep and try to uncover and provide for another person's. Well-supported and reflective teamwork can often help to redefine a 'behaviour' from one that is challenging to one that is an opportunity for improved well-being.

Cultures in which it is normal to *constantly look to make things better, help people to enjoy places where they spend time* and *help people to be active in a way that fulfils them every day* also help to not only make response to distress easier, but also prevent their likelihood in the first place. If it is normal for us to think about the environment's impact, to avoid boredom for people and to change what we do in response to a person's needs then many of the underlying causes of behaviour are removed through this positive action.

Here, a resident's niece reflected on how the staff's approach made a big difference to her uncle's experience, especially as he had been labelled in previous environments as 'challenging':

> They don't look on him as somebody who has got the dementia, and so they treat him as if he's just normal and can think normal and do normal things, so that's really good... Sometimes they kneel down beside him, or they draw up a chair and they'll... hold his hand and talk him through whatever's going through his mind. When he first came...he'd say things like, 'Oh they're coming to murder me,' or 'They're coming to shoot me,' when he has flashbacks I think to the war years of things that happened. And he'd say, he'd like not criticise but he'd be afraid of one or two people, you know, residents and things, and [care workers would] just calm him down, almost making sure and say, 'Oh no, no that's not going to happen.'

Part 2 (page 201) provides questions to help you assess your organisation's performance on this indicator.

6. Advocacy: Do we speak out on behalf of people living with dementia to make sure their rights, respect and dignity are upheld?

The most difficult situations are when the rights of one individual are at odds with the safety and comfort of others. An example of this might arise within a housing facility where a tenant who is disorientated is knocking on neighbours' doors. Another example could be within a residential home where a resident has become sexually disinhibited and is making sexual advances to others that are not welcomed. In such a situation, the initial response is that the person who is causing the problem should be removed. The problem with this response is that it may actually exacerbate the problem for the individual concerned and simply make it someone else's responsibility. In some cases, it may truly be the case that the individual's needs can be better met elsewhere because of better trained staff, a more suitable environment or higher staffing ratios.

There is no simple solution to situations such as these, but they occur with enough regularity that some mechanism for dealing with them needs to be in place before they occur. This sort of situation usually gives rise to a case conference or case review, and the person who may not be able to argue their own corner should have someone advocating on their behalf. In some situations, this might be a social worker or a community nurse. In other situations, it might be that the organisation calls on the services of a formal advocacy service.

An organisational culture in which *we all matter to each other* can be very important in enabling advocacy and effective resolution of competing rights and situations. When people have a connection to and opportunities to be involved with the community of the organisation then their roles and sense of responsibility in making 'the community' work become clearer and easier to act upon. A sense of understanding and connection of others in that organisational community can help prevent the polarised, 'them and us' positions that can be very difficult to reconcile. This does not mean that problems disappear in connected communities but that connection creates opportunities to raise problems and find solutions at early stages and in a way that accepts the differing perspectives involved.

A culture in which *leadership protects front-line service delivery* in relation to external factors such as commissioning and assessment processes, multidisciplinary support and expectations from families and friends will also be in a better position to pre-empt problems and negotiate conflicting positions and needs in positive and proactive ways.

In this example, a relative reflected on the way her mum's care home had advocated for her mum to ensure she was in the right sort of environment as her needs changed and dementia progressed, even though the change was initially worrying for her family. The home had not only advocated for her mum but also found ways to ease her family's concerns and thus help a necessary transition. Leadership and front-line staff had worked together to make this happen:

I realised mum wasn't going down to [specialist unit]. I mentioned it to [the manager] and she said, 'Well really she needs to come up here now.' I was a bit upset about it because, as I say I thought mum belongs down in [specialist unit] and I know the staff all down there really well, but I've got to admit since coming up here she has improved, and I think it's because it's quieter. I've accepted it, I said to [Mum], 'You're very happy up here,'... The other week mum was joining in things, and they were so excited that they videoed her, and they have actually sent the video through to my computer.'

Part 2 (page 202) provides questions to help you assess your organisation's performance on this indicator.

Summary

Element 3 of person-centred care is about providing care that tries to look at life from the perspective of the person living with dementia. Care is provided in a way where the priority is placed on promoting the well-being of people with dementia. The degree to which organisations take the viewpoint of people with dementia seriously can be seen in reactions to distress, day-to-day communication, empathic ability of care staff and vigilance around physical health and advocacy.

6

Social Environment

Element 4 of person-centred care is providing a social environment that supports psychological needs

Providing a supportive social environment: recognising that all human life is grounded in relationships and that people living with dementia need an enriched social environment that both compensates for their impairment and fosters opportunities for personal growth.

Key indicators for the social environment

- **Inclusion**: Are people helped to feel part of what is going on around them and supported to participate in a way that they are able?

- **Respect**: Does the support we provide show people that they are respected as individuals with unique identities, strengths and needs?

- **Warmth**: Does the atmosphere we create help people to feel welcomed, wanted and accepted?

- **Validation**: Are people's emotions and feelings recognised, taken seriously and responded to?

- **Enabling**: Does the support we provide help people to be as active and involved in their lives as possible? Are people treated as equal partners in their care?

- **Part of the community**: Does our service do all it can to keep people connected with their local community and the local community connected with the service?

- **Relationships**: Do we know about, welcome and involve the people who are important to a person?

> How you relate to us has a big impact on the course of the disease. You can restore our personhood, and give us a sense of being needed and valued. There is a Zulu saying that is very true. 'A person is a person through others.' Give us reassurance, hugs, support, a meaning in life. Value us for what we can still do and be, and make sure we retain social networks. It is very hard for us to be who we once were, so let us be who we are now and realise the effort we are making to function. (Bryden 2005, p.127)

In providing person-centred care, a supportive and nurturing social environment is the key to maintaining personhood on a day-to-day basis. Personhood can only be maintained in the context of relationships. Carl Rogers saw relationships as key to therapeutic growth and change. He highlighted the importance of the relationship and therapeutic alliance in person-centred counselling. Tom Kitwood's view of person-centred care for people with dementia was that it took place in the context of relationships – *Person to Person* was the title of Kitwood and Bredin's (1992a) first book on person-centred dementia care in practice. John Bond also included the context of relationships within his description of personhood:

> …individuals do not function in isolation, they also have relationships with others; all human life is interconnected and interdependent. (Bond 2001, p.47)

The maintenance of relationships is not dependent on verbal skills. As Ian Morton (1999) said, as verbal abilities are lost, the importance of warm, accepting human contact through non-verbal channels becomes even more important. Also, people with dementia may be more aware of any incongruence in what is being communicated verbally and non-verbally, because of their stronger reliance on non-verbal communication. Steven Sabat's (2001) demonstration of social positioning with respect to people with dementia lent empirical support to the manner in which interactions enhance or diminish a person's sense of self. His work also provides evidence of the way people with dementia actively cope with how they are treated.

The importance of conceptualising the person with dementia in relationship to others has been underlined by the coining of the term 'relationship-centred care'. Mike Nolan (Nolan, Davies and Grant 2001) offers a very useful framework about conceptualising relationships in care homes based on developing a sense of security, continuity, belonging, purpose, achievement and significance. Obviously, this is of particular importance for an organisation such as a care home, in which people live for long periods of time and whose sense of community and being connected with the world will be highly reliant on that organisation. The importance of links between the care home and community, and the relationships within the home itself, has long been recognised as central to improving the lives of people who live, work and visit care homes, as evidenced by the My Home Life movement (Owen and Meyer 2012). However, the importance of this community also extends to other types of organisations whether people live or work in them, stay temporarily or visit them occasionally.

Maintaining personhood

Kitwood (1997a) wrote about what people with dementia need from those around them to enable them to feel like a person – to maintain personhood. He chose a flower with overlapping petals to illustrate these needs, with love being the central need in the heart of the flower. We adapted this flower diagram in Figure 2.1 (page 35) to show how person-centred organisation can support these needs being met. The love referred to here is an unconditional acceptance that is generous and forgiving and asks for no reward.

There are many care workers and professionals who can show love to the people they care for in this way. It does not need to be taught to them. Indeed, sometimes in our rush to become professional or expert, that initial motivation of loving care can get lost along the way.

> As we become more emotional and less cognitive, it's the way you talk to us, not what you say, that we will remember. We know the feeling, but don't know the plot. Your smile, your laugh and your touch are what we will connect with. Empathy heals. Just love us as we are. We're still here, in emotion and spirit, if only you could find us. (Bryden 2005, p.138)

Kitwood (1997a) identified five major psychological needs that, if they are met, can greatly help people's sense of personhood. Most care practitioners can recognise ways by which they can meet those needs and help to maintain personhood in our day-to-day work with people living with dementia.

Comfort

The first need is for comfort. This is the provision of warmth and closeness to others. Comfort is about the provision of tenderness, closeness and soothing. It promotes security and decreases anxiety. It helps people relax. Comfort can be provided through physical touch, or through comforting words or gestures. Comfort also includes physical comfort with one's body. A lack of comfort will be experienced by those who are in pain, who feel physically ill or unwell, or who are sitting or lying in an unpleasant place.

> My stress tolerance is very low, and even a minor disruption can cause a catastrophic reaction, where I shout or scream, panic and pace. I need calm, no surprises, no sudden changes. Anxiety is an undercurrent of our disease. I feel I have to do something but can't remember what and often it feels like something terrible is going to happen, but I have forgotten what it is. With the stress of many activities at once, I become very focused, trying with all the brain I have left to concentrate. Telling me to rest won't help, but helping me to complete the task will. (Bryden 2005, p.111)

Identity

This relates to the need to know who you are and how you feel about yourself. Often, as the recent memories fade and language becomes problematic, identity is increasingly provided by those around the person with dementia. Identity relates to knowing who one is and to having a sense of continuity with the past. It is also about having a life story that is held and maintained, either by the person with dementia, or for them by others. Others know about you, they know who you are and they hold you in esteem. Identity can be undermined, particularly if people sense they are being treated like a child or if someone feels labelled or told off. Identity is supported by being treated with respect and by warm acceptance.

> Please don't call us 'dementing' – we are still people separate from our disease, we just have a disease of the brain. If I had cancer you would not refer to me as 'cancerous' would you? (Bryden 2005, p.143)

> Helen said she often felt lost, even in her own home. It was not really a matter of losing her way, but losing herself somehow... Somehow in her head, there was no sense of being a person existing in this space. Helen said it was worse when she was by herself but when others related to her, she seemed to come back from somewhere where she had been lost. Maybe they acted like a mirror for her, reflecting her existence, reaffirming her personhood. (Bryden 2005, p.43)

Attachment

Human beings are a highly social species and need to feel attached to others, particularly at times of heightened anxiety and change. Attachment relates to bonding, connection, nurture, trust and relationship. It also relates to security in relationships, and feeling that one has trusted others to whom one can turn in times of trouble or need. When people are anxious, the need to feel attached to someone or something familiar often increases to a significant degree. Attachment needs can be supported by acknowledgement, genuineness and validation. Attachment can be undermined by accusations and by being fobbed off and having one's strong emotions belittled.

The future looks bleak to the person with dementia – it not only looks bleak, but actually is bleak so I believe it is wrong to deny us help to deal with the whole gamut of emotions we will experience along the journey of this disease. (Bryden 2005, p.131)

Try to enter our distorted reality, because if you make us fit in with your reality, it will cause us extra stress. (Bryden 2005, p.147)

Occupation

This relates to being involved in the process of life. It fulfils a deep need for individuals to have an impact on the world and those around them. Occupation relates to being involved in activity in a way that is personally meaningful. It also relates to having a sense of agency, which is about feeling one has control over the world and can make things happen. It is about feeling that one can have an effect and impact on what is done and how. Occupation is supported by empowering, enabling, facilitating and collaborative staff skills. Occupation is undermined by disempowerment, disruption, imposition and being treated like an inanimate object.

We feel as if we are hanging onto a high cliff, above a lurking black hole. Daily tasks are complex. Nothing is automatic anymore. Everything is as if we are first learning. You tell us that we have asked you that question before, but we have no recollection. It is just a blank for the past and this feels strange and scary, and yet you are frustrated with us. If we had an arm or a leg missing you would congratulate us on our efforts but you cannot see how much of our brain is missing and how hard it is to cope so you don't understand our struggles. (Bryden 2005, p.98)

Inclusion

Being part of a group is a deeply embedded human need related to survival. People living with dementia are at great risk of being socially isolated even when they live in a communal setting. If no effort is made to help people be included by others, it becomes increasingly unlikely that they will be able to manage this for themselves and a state of depression and vegetation may occur.

Inclusion is about being in or being brought into the social world, either physically or verbally. It relates to facilitating engagement where there would otherwise be none, and making a person feel they are part of the group and are welcomed and accepted. Recognising people's worth, including them in discussions and activities, emphasising a sense of belonging and having fun together all support the need for people to feel included. Stigmatising, ignoring, banishment and mockery undermine the need for inclusion being met.

> Your name – the label that belongs to you – often is not there. Your face is familiar somehow but meeting you happens too quickly for me to search through my disjointed memory and find a label for you or a context of why I know you. I need time and clues, not questions. Try to chat about shared experiences so that I can find out why I know you, then maybe your label will appear. I realised something quite important about the way I recognise people. I would see a face and know it well and there would be a spark of recognition, and of joy in knowing. I would then smile and hug these dear people for I knew they loved me for who I am. (Bryden 2005, p.109)

Malignant Social Psychology and Positive Person Work

As with all the elements of person-centred care, ensuring that people with dementia have the opportunity for social, supportive and loving relationships with all those around them seems so obvious that surely we do not need a set of guidelines to achieve it. However, an examination of care provision shows that this is often not the norm in many services for people living with dementia, whether in their own homes, receiving support in the community or living in long-term care. Malignant Social Psychology (MSP) and Positive Person Work (PPW) relate directly to the psychological needs that Kitwood identified. Kitwood's writing on MSP helps to clarify why this seems so difficult to achieve.

Kitwood (1997a) described personhood being undermined by MSP of care where people with dementia experience dehumanising interactions such as being stigmatised, invalidated and ignored. These MSP actions or behaviours are rarely created with any malicious intent; rather, they become woven into the culture of care. The impact of this on the well-being of people with dementia, who are already struggling to adapt to neurological impairment and to maintain their sense of self, is hypothesised as being highly psychologically damaging.

Kitwood also described what a positive social psychology might look like for people with dementia. If personhood is undermined by MSP then it should also be possible to describe the sorts of everyday interactions that would promote the maintenance of personhood. He used the term 'Positive Person Work' (PPW) to describe different forms of interaction that would help maintain personhood. These were labelled recognition, negotiation, collaboration, play, timalation (engagement through the senses), celebration, relaxation, validation, holding and facilitation (Kitwood 1997a, pp.90–3).

We have worked with these concepts for many years now, both in education and research and through developments within the eighth edition of *Dementia Care Mapping* where we linked different types of MSP and PPW to Kitwood's psychological needs (Brooker and Surr 2006). This has been translated into practical handbooks for communication for front-line care workers and families in the USA (Verity and Kuhn 2008) and Australia (McCarthy 2011).

These concepts help us to think about and work upon some of the cultural influences that might be at play and affect organisational behaviours. In Chapter 2 we discussed organisational culture and the role that 'norms of behaviour' (unquestioned ways of thinking, feeling and acting) play in reinforcing both positive and negative cultures. Remember, norms become established because they provide workable solutions to the problems, issues and challenges we face in our everyday work practice. They are so consistently witnessed and experienced that it is hard to break the habit or even see that there might be a different way of doing things. We almost become trapped in those habits as we respond to daily problems.

This is what Kitwood was describing when he explained MSP. If MSP is employed unthinkingly as a response to everyday problems and challenges of supporting people living with dementia, then we need actively to highlight it and find different, more person-centred ways of solving those everyday problems and challenges: This is PPW. By challenging yourself and others to practise a PPW approach to those everyday issues, you begin a cycle that, over time, transforms the culture itself.

We will discuss each of the MSP and PPW actions and behaviours in turn, providing examples of when they might occur and how they can enhance or detract from a person's well-being. A familiarity with these can be very useful when trying to establish what is contributing to the good or bad 'feeling' you have about an interaction or setting. We display them here in pairs, where a common MSP behaviour is contrasted with an action that is more in line with a PPW approach. They are not exact opposites and there are overlaps between different behaviours and responses. However, examining them in this way can help us to think of alternatives to long ingrained habits and practices.

The examples used here are ones we have commonly seen in our research and time spent in care and support services. They are also common dilemmas and situations explained to us by those working on the front line providing direct care and support to people with dementia in a variety of settings

Person's psychological need: Comfort	
MSP that detracts from need: Intimidation	**PPW that meets the need**: Warmth
Making a person fearful by using spoken threats or physical power.	Demonstrating genuine affection, care and concern for the person.
Scenario: Omar is visited every day by a district nurse to check and redress a wound. Omar finds it hard to understand the treatment, which can be painful. He will often shout out and push the nurse away.	
MSP response: The nurse stands over Omar and says, 'You have to have this done now, Omar. If you don't I'll have to tell the Doctor you're not complying with treatment, and he'll have you taken into hospital.'	**PPW response**: The nurse sits by Omar and explains what she is going to do, saying, 'I can see you're worried, I would be too, but you will feel more comfortable afterwards.' She puts his favourite CD on, and encourages Omar to sing along as she checks the wound.

Person's psychological need: Comfort	
MSP that detracts from need: Withholding	**PPW that meets the need**: Holding
Refusing to give asked-for attention or to meet an evident need for contact.	Providing safety, security and comfort to a person.
Scenario: On a busy hospital ward a patient (Mr Martin) cries out: 'Help me, help me, please help me.' Staff are very busy providing care and support for other patients on the ward.	
MSP response: A healthcare assistant turns to her colleague and says, 'He'll just have to wait his turn. We have to do Bed 4 next as the surgeon is coming soon.'	**PPW response**: The healthcare assistant asks her colleague to get started with the next patient. She kneels next to Mr Martin and holds his hand. 'Mr Martin, it's okay, I'm sorry we're so slow today,' she soothes him for a few minutes and then says, 'We will be with you by half past eight, keep an eye on the clock.' She then joins her colleague.

Person's psychological need: Comfort	
MSP that detracts from need: Outpacing	**PPW that meets the need**: Relaxed pace
Providing information and presenting choices at a rate that is too fast for the person.	Recognising the importance of helping to create a relaxed atmosphere.
Scenario: Mr Nadir is visiting the GP with his daughter to receive the results of some blood tests and discuss further treatment for severe anaemia.	
MSP response: The GP reads the results off the computer screen and recommends a course of treatment, handing Mr Nadir a prescription. When Mr Nadir says he hasn't ever had a blood test, the GP replies, 'Well, never mind, just take the tablets and I'll see you in a few weeks.'	**PPW response**: The GP encourages Mr Nadir and his daughter to book a double appointment, to create more time to explain. She explains why they undertook the blood tests and what the results were. Mr Nadir agrees that he is always feeling very tired. The GP explains that by taking the tablets she is prescribing, Mr Nadir should feel less tired. Mr Nadir agrees this would be a good idea.

Person's psychological need: Identity	
MSP that detracts from need: Infantilisation	**PPW that meets the need**: Respect
Treating a person in a patronising way, as if they were a child.	Treating the person as a valued member of the community and recognising their age and experience.
Scenario: Emily is eating a Sunday dinner at the table with several other residents. She eats quite slowly and needs a lot of prompting from staff.	
MSP response: The care worker sitting at the table points to her dinner plate and says, 'Come on sweetie pie, eat up, there's a good girl.'	**PPW response**: The care worker sitting at the table says, 'Emily, your sister told me you used to cook Sunday lunch for all the family, how do these roast potatoes compare to yours?' She prompts Emily to try some and see.

Person's psychological need: Identity	
MSP that detracts from need: Labelling	**PPW that meets the need**: Acceptance
Using a label or categorisation as a way to describe or relate to a person.	Entering into a relationship based on an attitude of acceptance or positive regard for the person.
Scenario: A manager is showing visitors around the day centre and explaining what happens each day. A member of the day centre, Annie, passes by several times, walking around the centre's corridors and chatting to herself.	
MSP response: The manager turns to the visitors as Annie passes by and says, 'That's Annie, she's one of our wanderers,' and then carries on the tour.	**PPW response**: The manager approaches Annie and says, 'Hello Annie, I'm showing these people around, would you like to walk with us?' When Annie continues on her own way, the manager turns to the visitors and says, 'That's Annie, we might meet her again in a little while.'

Person's psychological need: Identity	
MSP that detracts from need: Disparagement	**PPW that meets the need**: Celebration
Telling a person that he or she is incompetent, useless, worthless or incapable.	Recognising, supporting and taking delight in the skills and achievements of the person.

Scenario: A domiciliary care worker has prepared soup and a sandwich for Mr Santos. When she returns to the dining table, he has taken the sandwich apart and is dipping it in the soup. There is soup all over the table and sandwich on the floor.

MSP response: The care worker sighs and says, 'Look at the mess you've made. I can't leave you alone for five minutes.' She takes the bowl away and wipes the table with a dish cloth.	**PPW response**: The care worker comes over and says, 'You look like you're enjoying that! I love to dip bread in my soup too.' She returns to the kitchen and gets a cloth, ready for when Mr Santos has finished.

Person's psychological need: Attachment	
MSP that detracts from need: Accusation	**PPW that meets the need**: Acknowledgment
Blaming a person for things they have done, or have not been able to do.	Recognising, accepting and supporting the person as unique and valuing them as an individual.

Scenario: An activities worker takes two residents out to the shops. Mrs Anders tries on a pair of red shoes, but then becomes upset and angry when she cannot buy them because she does not have enough money. The activities worker needs to update staff on what happened when she returns.

MSP response: The activities worker says, 'I'm not taking her again. She got so jealous when Mrs Smith got to buy some new shoes. Getting her home was nightmare.'	**PPW response**: The activities worker says, 'We need to make sure Mrs Anders always has enough money when we go shopping. It was hard for her when she couldn't have shoes and Mrs Smith could.'

Person's psychological need: Attachment	
MSP that detracts from need: Treachery	**PPW that meets the need**: Genuineness
Using trickery or deception to distract or manipulate a person in order to make them do or not to do something.	Being honest and open with the person in a way that is sensitive to their needs and feelings.
Scenario: Mr Khan has been staying at a care home since his wife died a month ago. He regularly goes to the front door and asks to go home to see his wife. If the door is open he will head home, and if it's closed he'll ask someone to let him out.	
MSP response: A care assistant approaches Mr Khan and says, 'Your wife will be here soon. Why don't you have a cup of tea with us?' Mr Khan goes with him to have a cup of tea.	**PPW response**: A care assistant approaches Mr Khan and says, 'I can see you are quite worried Mr Khan, can I help?' When Mr Khan asks for his wife the worker says, 'You must be missing her, tell me about her.' The worker sits down with Mr Khan and his photo album, talking through pictures of his family.

Person's psychological need: Attachment	
MSP that detracts from need: Invalidation	**PPW that meets the need**: Validation
Failing to acknowledge the reality of a person in a particular situation.	Recognising and supporting the reality of the person. Showing sensitivity to their feelings and emotions as a priority.
Scenario: Christine has been taken to accident and emergency following a fall at home. She is in the waiting area sitting in a wheelchair and is shouting loudly that she is frightened and wants to go home.	
MSP response: The admitting nurse walks up to Christine and says, 'Please don't shout out like that, you're perfectly safe here. It won't get you treated any faster, you know.'	**PPW response**: The admitting nurse says, 'It's very noisy in here, isn't it? I'm not surprised you want to go home.' She then explains why Christine is waiting and positions Christine's wheelchair so that she can see the receptionist, who waves at her and steps out to remind her every so often why she is here.

Person's psychological need: Occupation	
MSP that detracts from need: Disempowerment	**PPW that meets the need**: Empowerment
Not allowing a person to use the abilities that they have.	Letting go of control and assisting the person to be involved, discover and use abilities and skills.
Scenario: Sally is living at home and receives support from visiting care workers twice a day to help make sure she eats regular meals and takes her medication. Sally loves cooking, but finds it hard to prepare a whole meal, as she can forget to do important steps.	
MSP response: When the care worker arrives she encourages Sally to sit in the lounge and watch TV whilst she prepares the food. She says it takes too long when Sally is in the kitchen.	**PPW response**: The care worker and Sally go to the kitchen together. The care worker gives step-by-step instructions to Sally and steps in if Sally appears confused. It takes longer, but it means that the second visit for the day can be shorter, as they prepare both meals in advance at the lunchtime visit.

Person's psychological need: Occupation	
MSP that detracts from need: Imposition	**PPW that meets the need**: Facilitation
Forcing a person to do something, overriding their own desires or wishes or denying them choices.	Assessing the level of support a person needs and providing it.
Scenario: After receiving personal care, Flo is rooting through her handbag and saying, 'Gotta find some lippy.'	
MSP response: The care assistant takes the bag off Flo and finds the lipstick, bends down and puts some on Flo's lips, before wheeling her out of the room and into the lounge.	**PPW response**: The care worker says, 'Well remembered, Flo. Can't leave without doing your face! Shall I find it for you?' She locates the lipstick, opens it and hands it to Flo, 'I'll just get you a mirror, Flo.'

Person's psychological need: Occupation	
MSP that detracts from need: Disruption	**PPW that meets the need**: Enabling
Intruding or interfering with something the person is doing or crudely breaking their frame of reference.	Recognising and encouraging a person's level of engagement within their frame of reference.
Scenario: Several attendees at a day centre are sitting at a table together and painting. Jeff takes the paintbrush from the tub and starts to rub it on his trousers.	
MSP response: A support worker takes the paintbrush from Jeff saying, 'Don't do it like that, here let me show you.'	**PPW response**: A support worker says, 'Are you getting the crumbs off those Jeff? Looking very smart.' He uses his own brush to make a mark on the paper so Jeff can see how it's done.

Person's psychological need: Occupation	
MSP that detracts from need: Objectification	**PPW that meets the need**: Collaboration
Treating a person as if they were an object, or a lump of meat.	Treating a person as a full and equal partner in what is happening. Consulting and working with them.
Scenario: A resident in a care home, Lilly, needs support to eat as she has very poor control over her hand movements.	
MSP response: A staff member sits next to Lilly and spoons food towards her mouth saying, 'Open,' every so often.	**PPW response**: A staff member sits next to Lilly and says, 'What do you want next on the fork?' Lilly points, 'Potato? Want some gravy as well?' Lilly nods.

Person's psychological need: Inclusion	
MSP that detracts from need: Stigmatisation	**PPW that meets the need**: Recognition
Treating a person as if they are an outcast, alien or a diseased object.	Meeting the person in their own uniqueness, bringing an open and prejudiced attitude.

Scenario: Ms Edison arrives for her GP appointment but is confused by a computerised log-in system. After a while she goes to the reception desk and says she is here for an appointment.

MSP response: The receptionist sighs heavily and tells Ms Edison to use the computer. When Ms Edison says that she doesn't understand it the receptionist rolls her eyes and says under her breath, 'Here we go again,' before telling Ms Edison to sit down, as she is causing a queue.	**PPW response**: The receptionist smiles at Ms Edison and says, 'Hello, how can I help you?' When she finds out Ms Edison's name she tells her that she'll let the doctor know and to take a seat in the waiting room. When Ms Edison hesitates the receptionist gets up to show her to a seat, saying, 'We've changed everything around since you were last here, I think.'

Person's psychological need: Inclusion	
MSP that detracts from need: Ignoring	**PPW that meets the need**: Including
Carrying on (in action or conversation) in the presence of a person as if they are not there.	Enabling and encouraging the person to be involved and feel included, both physically and psychologically.

Scenario: Two members of staff are discussing the rota for the following day when a patient comes up to the desk, bangs it and says, 'Will Mary be coming, do you think?'

MSP response: The staff say to the patient, 'We're on about staff not visitors,' and then turn their chairs away from the desk so their backs are to the patient. The patient walks away.	**PPW response**: The staff look up at the patient and say, 'I'm not sure about Mary. Do you think you could help us out?' They pull up an extra chair and the patient holds the rota sheet while the staff continue planning.

Person's psychological need: Inclusion	
MSP that detracts from need: Banishment	**PPW that meets the need**: Belonging
Sending a person away or excluding them physically or psychologically.	Providing a sense of acceptance in a particular setting, regardless of abilities or disabilities.
Scenario: Mr Klein visits a day centre every day. He can support himself to eat, although he can get very messy when he does it. Some of the fellow centre attendees have complained about having to sit near him, as it puts them off their food.	
MSP response: The support workers discuss it and decide to sit Mr Klein in the corner of the lunchroom facing away from others, as they agree it's not very nice to look at.	**PPW response**: The support workers ask Mr Klein where he would like to sit for lunch and when he has taken his place, if no other attendees sit near him, a worker takes their lunch and sits next to him, keeping him company.

Person's psychological need: Inclusion	
MSP that detracts from need: Mockery	**PPW that meets the need**: Fun
Making fun of a person; teasing, humiliating them and making jokes at their expense.	Accessing a free and creative way of being, and using and responding to the use of fun and humour.
Scenario: Marjory lives in a residential home and likes to get herself dressed in the morning, but quite often forgets items of clothing. One morning she comes into the communal lounge wearing a thin petticoat. She twirls in it and shows it to several other residents.	
MSP response: Several care workers giggle as she walks in saying, 'Here she goes again, showing off her nicks!' At handover they recount the story calling her an 'exhibitionist'.	**PPW response**: A support worker comes over to Marjory and says, 'What a lovely petticoat you have there Marjory, perfect for dancing in, can I join you?' She dances with Marjory towards the corner of the room and then whispers to her, 'Shall I help you get the skirt on over the top?'

What it might feel like to have personhood undermined or supported

Below are two pieces of prose taken from *Dementia Reconsidered* by Tom Kitwood (1997a). The first is imagining what the internal world might feel like for a person with dementia living in a care setting where personhood is undermined.

You are in a swirling fog, and in half-darkness. You are wandering around in a place that seems vaguely familiar; and yet you do not know where you are; you cannot make out whether it is summer or winter, day or night. At times the fog clears a little, and you can see a few objects really clearly; but as soon as you start to get your bearings, you are overpowered by a kind of dullness and stupidity; your knowledge slips away, and again you are utterly confused.

While you are stumbling in the fog, you have an impression of people rushing past you, chattering like baboons. They seem to be so energetic and purposeful, but their business is incomprehensible. Occasionally you pick up fragments of conversation, and have the impression that they are talking about you. Sometimes you catch sight of a familiar place; but as you move towards the face it vanishes, or turns into a demon. You feel desperately lost, alone, bewildered and frightened. In this dreadful state you find that you cannot control your bladder, or your bowels; you are completely losing your grip; you feel dirty, guilty, ashamed; it's so unlike how you used to be, that you don't even know yourself.

And then there are the interrogations. Official people ask you to perform strange tasks which you cannot fully understand; such as counting backwards from one hundred, or obeying the instruction 'if you are over 50 put your hands above your head'. You are never told the purpose or the results of these interrogations. You'd be willing to help, eager to co-operate, if only you knew what it was all about, and if someone took you seriously enough to guide you.

This is present reality: everything is falling apart, nothing gets completed, nothing makes sense. Behind the fog and the darkness there is a vague memory of good times, when you knew where and who you were, when you felt close to others, and when you were able to perform daily tasks with skill and grace; once the sun shone brightly and the landscape of life had richness and pattern. But now all that has been vandalised, ruined, and you are left in chaos, carrying the terrible sense of loss that can never be made good. Once you were a person who counted; now you are nothing, and good for nothing. A sense of oppression hangs over you, intensifying at times into naked terror; its meaning is that you might be abandoned forever, left to rot and disintegrate into un-being.

Taken from Kitwood, T. (1997a) Dementia Reconsidered. Buckingham:
Open University Press, p. 77. [1]

The second is what life could be like if care was truly person-centred.

You are in a garden, at the start of a summer's day. The air is warm and gentle, carrying the sweet scent of flowers, and a slight mist is floating around. You can't make out the shape of everything, but you are aware of some beautiful colours, blue, orange, pink and purple; the grass is green as emerald. You don't know where you are, but this doesn't matter. You somehow feel 'at home', and there is a sense of harmony and peace.

As you walk around, you become aware of other people. Several of them seem to know you; it is a joy to be greeted so warmly, and by name. There are one or two of them whom you feel sure you know well. And then there is that one special person. She seems so warm, so kind, so understanding. She must be your mother; how good it is to be back with her again. The flame of life now burns brightly and cheerfully within you. It hasn't always been like this. Somewhere, deep inside, there are dim memories of times of crushing loneliness and ice-cold fear. When that was, you do not know; perhaps it was in another life. Now there is company whenever you want it, and quietness when that is what you prefer. This is the place where you belong, with these wonderful people; they are like a kind of family.

The work that you do here is the best that you have ever had. The hours are flexible, and the job is pleasant; being with people is what you have always enjoyed. You can do the work at exactly your own pace, without any rush or pressure, and you can rest whenever you need. For instance there is a kind man who often comes to see you – by a strange coincidence his name is the same as that of your husband. He seems to need you, and to enjoy being with you. You, for your part, are glad to give time to being with him, his presence, strangely, gives you comfort.

---

1   This material is reproduced with the kind permission of The Open University Press/McGraw-Hill Publishing Company.

As you pass a mirror you catch a glimpse of a person who looks quite old. Is it your grandmother or that person who used to live next door? Anyway, it is good to see her too. Then you begin to feel tired: you find a chair and you sit down, alone. Soon you become aware of a chill around your heart, a sinking feeling in your stomach – the deadly fear is coming over you again. You are about to cry out, but then you see that kind mother-person, already there, sitting beside you. Her hand is held out towards you, waiting for you to grasp it. As you talk together, the fear evaporates like the morning mist, and you are again in the garden, relaxing in the golden warmth of the sun. You know it isn't heaven itself, but sometimes it feels as if it might be half way there.

Taken from Kitwood, T. (1997a) Dementia Reconsidered. Buckingham: Open University Press, pp. 84–5.[2]

Putting supportive social environments into practice

As with the personal perspectives element, the indicators in the supportive social environment element of VIPS primarily need to be led by those who are responsible for the day-to-day management of direct support staff and the direct service environment. These indicators are about the way in which direct support staff respond to those they care for and the skills and values they have in their communication with service users.

As in the last chapter, having responsibility for the direct day-to-day management of a service, or leading shifts within a service, is a tough job, and prioritising the interpersonal care is a real challenge when there are so many other competing calls on your time. However, having a sense about where you are now and where would you like to be in the future, and what might stand in your way can be helpful in taking small steps towards progress.

What follows is a series of questions to help your organisation benchmark where you are in terms of the supportive social environments element of person-centred care and consider the ways in which the organisational culture may enhance or challenge the achievement of it.

---

2   This material is reproduced with the kind permission of The Open University Press/McGraw-Hill Publishing Company.

1. Inclusion: Are people helped to feel part of what is going on around them and supported to participate in a way in which they are able?

In some care services, people with dementia are seen as part of the furniture – to be vacuumed around, tidied up and polished but not to be included or communicated with. They are 'done to' rather than involved in what is going on. This is true in many service settings where people are cared for, let alone those service settings for people with dementia. Think about the way that people waiting to be seen in accident and emergency departments are known as 'chairs', or people waiting to be discharged from hospital are 'bed-blockers'.

In order for people to get their needs for attachment and inclusion met, those providing support will often need to play an active role in ensuring that people are encouraged to take part in the social network of life. Staff have an active role in helping someone feel included on many levels. This might be by physically helping them move to somewhere where they can see others and be at the centre of the action, or it might be in knowing key stories from their life and prompting their use in conversation. It could involve encouraging the person to participate in the work and action that takes place in the service, such as helping the staff with collecting laundry.

Inclusion is facilitated (or restricted) by organisational culture in the following ways. Primarily, the extent to which people living with dementia are encouraged to be *active in a way that fulfils them every day* will make a huge difference to inclusion. Where involving people in ways that are meaningful to them to give them purpose and activity throughout the day is seen regularly and understood to be a fundamental part of everyone's work, inclusion becomes an expectation of every aspect of work in the home. In addition, knowing *we all matter to each other* can really help inclusion to occur because it ensures that everyone is known throughout the organisation, and everyone feels that they have a role to play in supporting the person. So, whether the member of staff is a cleaner, a doctor, the manager or a healthcare assistant, they know that part of their role is to support the person to feel included by engaging with them in the best way that they can.

In this example a care worker showed exceptionally skilled communication to include a resident who spent most of her day walking through the care home, rarely connecting with others:

> Betty comes down the corridor and the care worker smiles at her. Betty smiles back and lifts her arms in a dancing way. This is the most spontaneously animated I have seen her. The care worker smiles again and says, 'You okay?' He taps the seat and Betty sits down in chair next to him at the computer. He notices the old tissue in her hand and says, 'I'll get you a new one, come on.' He holds her hand, helps her stand, and walks slightly ahead to kitchen. He gives Betty a new tissue, 'I'll take that one, you have this one.'

This very tailored and attentive approach was also shown to a gentleman who spent most of his time alone in his bedroom, rarely venturing into the company of others.

> Care worker is sat by the computer, doing notes and listening to Graeme. He occasionally says, 'Yeah?' to prompt Graeme and keep him talking. Care worker says, 'Not busy today then?' It always sounds like he knows what Graeme is talking about. It's respectful and like they're peers. 'How's today been?' He asks Graeme, 'How's the football?' Graeme starts chatting about football, 'Who do you support?'

Part 2 (page 204) provides questions to help you assess your organisation's performance on this indicator.

2. Respect: Does the support we provide show people that they are respected as individuals with unique identities, strengths and needs?

Treating a person with respect and courtesy indicates a powerful message that we see the person as a valued member of society and that we hold them in esteem. We enter into a relationship with someone we respect based on an attitude of acceptance and positive regard. We recognise them, remember them, take delight in their skills and celebrate achievements.

When this respect does not exist, tendencies towards patronising or dismissive attitudes will emerge in which people are told off, put down or their feelings and wishes disparaged. In an atmosphere of no respect, a person's shortcoming or difficulties will be labelled and will come to identify the person above all else: 'a wanderer' or 'a screamer'.

If people feel respected, they are more likely to show respect for themselves and for those around them. This is true for people living with dementia and for those supporting them. In a care organisation, how do front-line staff feel? Do they feel that their manager and organisation respects them as unique individuals with strengths and feelings? If the answer is no, then it will be hard to create a respectful culture overall.

A respectful approach is cultivated by an organisational culture that *empowers and supports front-line staff.* This is because empowerment comes through recognition and utilisation of people's strengths and support for their needs. When staff feel respected, they will have more capacity to support people living with dementia in similar ways. If they are not empowered in this way, then staff have to draw solely on their personal reserves to demonstrate and enact respect for people. This is emotionally draining, and over time or in stressful situations is unsustainable for even the most well-meaning and responsible person.

We *all work together to deliver the best care* is also crucial to sustaining a respectful culture, because it ensures that respect is thought about and demonstrated in a concrete way and that all understand it as part of the responsibilities. *We all matter to each other* helps to facilitate this respect because it means people understand how their behaviour affects others and undertake responsibility for thinking about how others may feel or perceive situations.

In this exchange, during a very busy period in the care home, we can see a sensitive and respectful interaction with a resident who may have needed support with personal care, but often found this a very distressing occurrence:

> Gary comes over to the medication trolley, where the lead carer is. He is pulling at his loose trousers. The lead carer chats to him about getting him a belt for Christmas. Another care worker comes over and says, 'You look very smart.' The lead carer then talks about dinner, 'Can I steal a few chips, Gary?' Gary replies, 'I won't tell anyone.' They both smile and laugh. 'Gary, do you want something? Is it the bathroom? Let me get someone to help you.' Bridget calls over another care worker and the care worker puts her hand on Gary's shoulder and says, 'I'll come and help you.'

Part 2 (page 205) provides questions to help you assess your organisation's performance on this indicator.

3. Warmth: Does the atmosphere we create help people to feel welcomed, wanted and accepted?

Showing warmth and unconditional positive regard is at the heart of a supportive social psychology that helps people to feel comfortable, confident and at ease. If people do not feel welcomed and wanted by those around them, then their personhood shrivels. It is so important for a person with dementia, because dementia reduces the ability to remind oneself of times when warmth has been shown or to interpret what is going on and how best to respond to that. If people feel unwelcome, a very natural reaction is to leave that place for somewhere where they will feel more welcome. If the person leaves the GP surgery before their appointment, their health might deteriorate further. If a person living with dementia tries to leave a hospital or care home, they will often be prevented from doing so and labelled us as 'escaping' or a 'wanderer'.

Is the service provision marked by smiles, welcome, genuine concern and helpfulness? Do staff demonstrate affection, care and concern for people they support and those who are important to them? Are people's calls for attention ignored or dismissed? Are information and choices presented at a rate that is too fast? Do we rely on systems, technology or signage that is hard to interpret and get impatient when people ask for help or do not do what is expected? Confrontation is another common response by front-line staff who do not understand the nature of dementia or who are working in a culture where blame and criticism are experienced regularly. Warmth is a far more likely action when dementia is properly understood, as staff have the knowledge to compensate for the damage in a person's brain through their own responses. Staff who experience warmth in response to their stresses and anxieties will be emotionally equipped to provide it in response to others' needs.

A social environment that demonstrates warmth is possible in a culture that *empowers and supports front-line staff* to take action on behalf of the people they support. Again, as with a social environment of respect, this requires that front-line staff are supported both practically and emotionally to deliver that warmth and to receive it themselves. Warmth also requires that staff *constantly look to make things better* for the people they care for and help people to be *active in a way that fulfils them every day.*

Knowing that *we all matter* will also create an atmosphere of warmth. This is because it helps everyone in the community to understand the role they can play and the impact they have (both positively and negatively) on others. *Leadership protecting front-line service delivery* is also important here and this may be particularly relevant for supporting families and visitors. Leadership and front-line managers will need to meet families' needs and anxieties with warmth, rather than simply delegating this responsibility to front-line staff. Without leadership taking responsibility for this there is a risk that staff can be left to try to meet the needs of both family/friends and the person living with dementia. This can be very difficult to do simultaneously, as at times people's needs can be contradictory. For example, it can be challenging to see your dad behaving in a way that appears very different to the person you know. This experience can bring anxieties and grief, which need to be met with warmth and understanding. However, good care for Dad also requires that his needs are met with warmth and understanding and this demands that front-line staff connect with him *as he is now.* This sort of situation requires careful attention and management from an entire staff team to ensure that both sets of needs are met with that warmth.

In this example, a resident is regularly standing during a mealtime and walking over to other residents, who appear to be getting annoyed. The care worker uses warmth to help the person take part in the mealtime and avoid too much disturbance of others.

> Each time [she stood up] a carer came and smiled warmly, sometimes engaging her with talk about her clothes and encouraged her back to her (nearest) seat, brought her meal and encouraged her to eat. The resident appeared to be easily agitated but appeared soothed by the carer. The carer had to repeatedly encourage the person to sit down and to spend some time eating [but] each time was like the first time; warm, smiling and as if pleased to be with the resident.

Part 2 (page 206) provides questions to help you assess your organisation's performance on this indicator.

4. Validation: Are people's emotions and feelings recognised, taken seriously and responded to?

Validation is the recognition and the supporting of the subjective reality of another person and having particular sensitivity to the feelings and emotional state of that person. There needs to be a genuine effort to understand and acknowledge the feelings of people receiving support. Their emotional state should be accepted and people not blamed or made to feel stupid for the way they feel.

If people feel that their emotional needs are respected and understood, they are more likely to be in a state of better emotional well-being over time. If distress is met promptly and empathically then it is likely to dissipate more quickly than if people spend long periods of time in unattended emotional distress.

In similar ways to warmth, a validating approach requires an organisational culture that *empowers and supports front-line staff* through provision of day-to day practical and emotional support. Empowered staff are able to take responsibility for discovering and responding to the emotional state of a person. However, if they are not skilled enough to pick up on those states, or are not able to effect any action in response, then validation becomes highly unlikely or reliant entirely on a staff member's own personal resources.

The three norms of care also help to embed validation, because they create an expectation that *staff will constantly look to make things better* and they will *help a person to enjoy places where they spend time* in order to respond to someone's emotional reality. When we expect people will be *active in a way that fulfils them every day* then, attentiveness to what is meaningful to a person's well-being occurs. These three norms of care also require that a manager can protect *front-line service delivery* as paramount so that the focus of their work is on attending to a person's needs rather than needs of the organisation, paperwork, finance, regulation etc.

> In this example, we see how important it is that staff are able to act on their empathy with someone's emotions and experiences to validate them and reinforce positive experiences. It also shows how staff can often be left in an intolerable bind if their ability to validate and respond is restricted by other forces:
>
>> Fred was a gentleman living with dementia, who became very distressed during personal care. This presented a great deal of physical challenges for his care workers, including being physically hurt at times. His key worker, in particular, showed a great deal of insight into how frightening and embarrassing personal care must be for a gentleman as independent and confused as Fred. She then talked about a difficulty they experienced when shaving Fred:
>>
>>> [It was easier to use face clippers rather than a razor] because sometimes he won't let me shave him for like two weeks, and it's that long, if I use a razor, it hurts him. But I'm just trying to keep on top of it as much as I can, because obviously without the face clippers it's hard. He got bought like some face clippers instead of, like the shaver, but it broke, and now his family are refusing to buy a new one because of how expensive they are, and the home won't buy one. So if I buy one I'm not going to get my money back. So it's a bit… I keep looking like to see if there's any deals or that, because I don't mind paying £10 out of my own money if it's going to make life, I don't know. But…the first one broke and then the second one just went missing. It's just one of those things.

> Part 2 (page 207) provides questions to help you assess your organisation's performance on this indicator.

5. Enabling: Does the support we provide help people to be as active and involved in their lives as possible? Are people treated as equal partners in their care?

Enabling means identifying and encouraging someone's level of engagement within their frame of reference. It is very easy in busy environments to take over a person with dementia completely: to feed them, to dress them and to wash them without enabling them to do the parts of these routines that they can for themselves. Not allowing people to use the abilities that they have is disempowering in the extreme.

The amount of support that individuals need with their own care will vary over time. The right amount of support will enable someone to feel empowered. Too little support will result in people feeling anxious and overwhelmed. Too much support can make people feel angry and stupid. The staff skills of facilitation – assessing the level of support required and providing the right amount – and collaboration – treating someone as a full and equal partner in what is happening, consulting and working with them – are critical if enabling is to occur.

At the extreme are environments where people are actively disabled by their surroundings. In these situations a person's wish to do something is overridden by others or thwarted by the environment. This can arise sometimes with people who walk for long periods of time. Where this is seen as a behaviour ('wandering') to be stopped, front-line staff's approach and the physical environment is used to constrain and prevent the behaviour, sometimes in highly restrictive and inappropriate ways. However, where it is seen as an expression of need and an ability the person still has, then the response becomes focused on meeting the need and facilitating the person's ability in a safe way.

There will be occasions when the risk of falling or danger is so high that a plan of care has to be in place to protect the well-being of that person. However, restraint, whether physical or chemical, should be a last resort and an option only used in the context of an approach that recognises the need to balance concerns about risk against the positive impact that taking risks has on a person's well-being. This need for an empowering approach is addressed within Chapter 5's indicator 'empathy and acceptable risk'.

Enabling and empowerment of people with dementia requires an organisational culture that *empowers and supports front-line staff* to take responsibility for day-to-day decision-making on behalf of the people they support. This is because staff need to have the freedom to act in response to people's changing abilities. Norms of care help embed an enabling approach because we expect *activity that fulfils every day* means a person's abilities are noted and enhanced. A care culture where staff *constantly look to make things better* for the people and provide *enjoyable places where they spend time* again ensures that situations constantly adapt to the needs of a person with supporters stepping back or stepping in as required.

In the following observation, a care worker is seen using tremendous skill and patience to help a resident (Britta) take a number of different medications. In total, this exchange lasted 15 minutes:

> The care worker says to Britta, 'This is to wash the tablets down, put these in your mouth and then have that.' It's a very patient exchange. Britta sips slowly and then says, 'It's a bit too much.' The care worker responds, 'I know, but the good news is that when it's gone you'll feel better because it's for your waterworks.' She chats about her dog with Britta and then puts the glass to her lips again and says, 'Just a little left.' Britta takes a sip. The care worker then says, 'Oooooh, now this one is your favourite!' Britta starts to sing and the care worker laughs. She puts the tablets in Britta's mouth. Britta turns her head, stops and starts to chat again. The care worker puts her head on Britta's shoulder, smiles and mirrors her facial expression. The care worker pops a tablet to Britta's lips again. Britta opens her mouth and takes it, 'You are absolutely excellent! Marvellous, all down the hatch.'

Part 2 (page 208) provides questions to help you assess your organisation's performance on this indicator.

6. Part of the community: Does our service do all it can to keep people connected with their local community and the local community connected to the service?

Although many of the large institutions where people with dementia lived for many years have closed down in the UK to be replaced with community facilities, the lived experience of institutionalisation survives. We still see too much service provision that requires the person to adapt their lives around what is available from the 'service provider' to the detriment of their involvement in their communities and everyday lives. A one-off appointment from a district nurse or care worker that gets in the way of regular routines may not be harmful, but when they regularly disrupt familiar routines and social networks then people's social community is broken down very quickly. Likewise, services that support people in their own homes are often seen as a 'sitting service' rather than as support that enables people to remain part of their community.

Within residential services, the idea of the closed institution where people never leave the building or grounds remains. Many people never get to put on a hat, coat and outdoor shoes, go on a bus or visit the pub, shop or place of worship. These are the activities that people take as part of ordinary life. They help us to maintain our identity and our interest in life in all its variety. People with dementia need this variety as much as anyone else.

In addition, the need for local communities to engage and step inside the care homes, day services and hospitals that exist within them is also important. Some places are still seen as if they have the large brick walls built around them that used to surround the old asylums. Places that encourage visitors also encourage life. There are many innovative schemes of therapists, artists and hobbyists visiting services. There is much that can be done by local friends and volunteers. Having a café that is open to people from outside, or a nursery or play scheme sharing some of the communal facilities, can help people maintain a sense of involvement in ordinary life and break down some of the stigma surrounding dementia.

We all matter to each other is a central feature of positive care cultures and without it a positive culture is impossible to sustain, because a sense of belonging and ownership of what goes on in the service cannot be built and people involved pull towards different ends instead of working together. The internal aspects of that connectivity are helped significantly by the external connection to the local community because the openness and input from outside in the form of volunteers, visitors etc. provide new opportunities and inspiration. If a care home, housing scheme or day service is well connected to its external community, it becomes a place that is understood and accepted; a place that is understood and accepted in turn becomes somewhere it is desirable to work in, live in and visit.

This example shows the importance of bringing the outside community into the care home. An activities worker explained about a recent visit by a donkey sanctuary to the home:

> Yeah, and they just went round, people weren't sure, you know, 'Oh let me take your hand,' so they're very good at interacting, knowing how, reading people. Like, 'If you put your hand on mine we can do it together.' This pony or whatever put their head in their lap. They have never seen anything like it. And I got the best buzz because a senior member of staff says, 'That is the best thing we've ever had in the 10 years.' I thought, 'Oh thanks,' so we'll do it again.

Equally, in this example, the importance of maintaining links with the outside world was discussed by an activities coordinator:

> We went out on Saturday. I just did it voluntary, we went out to hear the Choral Society singing the Messiah, and we took 15 of them on the minibus. And just to see them there, singing, crying, and coming home in the bus, it's one of the few times, it was just buzzing in the back of the bus, they were all talking to each other. And although it was hard work getting them there, and when we got there it was a mile and three lifts and all that to get them into the room, it was just worth it to see the pleasure when we got back, you know, and just what it had meant to them.

Part 2 (page 209) provides questions to help you assess your organisation's performance on this indicator.

7. Relationships: Do we know about, welcome and involve the people who are important to a person?

The onset of dementia can be likened to a storm that threatens a person's relationships. Just like any major health or life event, it challenges and puts pressures on those close to a person. It can also change the ways in which a person can contribute to a relationship through their own actions and this takes time and support for everyone to adapt to: Mum may have been the central hub of the family, negotiating between siblings and preventing arguments but if she is now less able to remember conversations and needs support from others, the dynamics and interactions change and this affects everybody involved. When providing support to a person, we must understand and accept that respecting and facilitating important relationships is part and parcel of person-centred care. We cannot care well for a person with dementia unless we also care well for those relationships that are important to them, however complex those relationships may be.

However, too often, families and friends are viewed in a negative light and talked of in terms that are just as labelling and stigmatising as those used to describe dementia itself. In addition, they are often conceived of in very narrow terms: as only the person's 'next of kin', children or most regular visitor, rather than all of the people who may be important and play different roles in someone's life. Our friends (both near and distant, past and present) are as important to our well-being as family members. Each of us has complex family relationships that vary considerably in terms of size, make-up and history. We have families by blood, step-families and families of choice, of which the latter may be more significant to our well-being. Our relationships are complex, ever changing and frequently challenging, but this only emphasises their importance to our identities and well-being.

When providing support to a person with dementia in any setting or service, our involvement can protect or fail to protect those relationships from the impact of dementia. All too often, support services can inadvertently become a bolt of lightning in the storm of dementia, placing additional pressures, demands and expectations on already frazzled relationships. Instead, we should be seeking to act as an umbrella under which the person and their important relationships can shelter by providing support, information and working in partnership with others.

How do we seek to find out about and involve people's significant friends and family? Are we careful to avoid imposing our own values and assumptions about what family 'should' be and do on another person with a unique history and set of relationships? How do we let people know that it is okay to be as involved or uninvolved as is possible for them? Do we consider the language and approaches we use to ensure we are not inadvertently alienating someone from a different culture or a person who may be gay, lesbian, bisexual or transgender? Do we help people to try and form new relationships through chances for conversation, hobbies and activities? This is particularly important in older age when bereavements can sharply shrink a person's social contacts.

Working positively with people's relationships is facilitated by a culture in which *we all matter to each other*. This is because that community provides opportunities for everyone to be involved in a variety of different ways and so suits whatever is right for that person's significant others at different times. Moreover, it helps to develop new relationships within the community, because staff and family members recognise their connection through the person with dementia and the person with dementia is recognised and accepted by others who are part of that community too. Connectedness also helps people to see others' values and skills. A person's oldest friend has a lot to give in terms of life history information, which can be invaluable to support staff. In turn, those staff have skills and knowledge of dementia and how to support the person as their needs change that the oldest friend may well be grateful for.

The cultural feature *we all work together* is also significant here because it can help everyone, whether support staff, family or friends, to understand and share the aim of person-centred care and contribute in ways that best suit their skills. Without constant work towards a consensus on what enhances a person's well-being, it is easy for services, staff and family members to have different goals and work at cross purposes.

In this example, a relative recalls an important interaction with staff in the early days of her mum's move into residential care that helped enhance important relationships:

> I remember when Mum first came in, I was sat…with her and she was having a bad day. And there was no one else around, there was just Mum and myself in the main lounge, and I couldn't get anything out of Mum and the tears were coming, you know. And one of the carers, I don't know where he came from but he put his hand on my shoulder, squeezed it and said, 'I know – are you alright?'
>
> And by golly that made such a difference, knowing that they cared not just for Mum but for the family as well. And I found that very warming, and within minutes I'd got a cup of tea in my hand and, no fuss made you know, I mean I felt a right idiot but in no way was I made to feel silly or belittled. But I just felt I was given that uplift and the support that I then needed. And I shall never forget that little act, because although in itself it was probably just everyday for him, it meant so much to me.

Part 2 (page 210) provides questions to help you assess your organisation's performance on this indicator.

Summary

Element 4 of person-centred care is about providing care that supports people in relationships with others, and helps them to remain part of the human club and involved in life. The lived experience of care is one where people feel secure, welcomed, validated and enabled through good communication and inclusive practice. Services are part of the community in its truest sense rather than mini institutions.

7

Care in Context

The term 'person-centred care' was first used by Kitwood (1988) to differentiate ways of working with people with dementia that were not framed within a biological or technical model. Understanding and expertise in the provision of person-centred care have developed enormously since the term was first used. The first edition of this book was an attempt to articulate the different elements of person-centred care and to describe what these look like in practice. We recognised that leadership at different levels within the care organisation have responsibilities and influence at different aspects of person-centred care. Within this second edition we want to underline this further still in acknowledging the importance of developing a strong care culture in which the different VIPS elements can flourish.

Ideally, all the VIPS elements work together. Sometimes this occurs by chance or unintentionally. For example, this may be the case in smaller care organisations where a leader with a strong person-centred value base communicates their vision throughout the whole team and a positive care culture emerges. The positive care culture sustains over time as new staff are employed who quickly learn the way of working. We might also surmise that a strong person-centred value base means that staff turnover is lower. This in turn helps to cement the positive care culture for the long term. However, even in these smaller organisations, this is not always the case and it is dangerous to assume that it will automatically occur.

Developing and maintaining a positive care culture in a larger care provider or across a number of care services is unlikely to occur simply by chance. To ensure that care remains person-centred requires leadership at all levels within the organisation to be in alignment. The VIPS elements and indicators provide this strategy. They provide a blueprint for helping care organisations to be clear about 'what good looks like'.

It is interesting to consider whether this definition might work as a model to facilitate some predictions of what might happen if only certain elements of person-centred care are in place while others are neglected. The following observations are based on experience of working with many care providers for people living with dementia. In addition, they help to illustrate the interconnection of the features of positive care cultures as discussed in Chapter 2. They are summarised diagrammatically in Table 7.1.

Table 7.1 All the VIPS elements need to work together

Lack of strength for this element	Element	Strength only in this element but not others
Discrimination against people with dementia and those who care for them. People with dementia do not have access to good-quality care.	**Valuing**	Care evangelism. Platitudes that people agree with but don't know how to put into practice. Glossy brochures but no substance.
Chaotic and inappropriate assessments and care plans for people with complex needs and life histories. Lack of continuity and integration of care.	**Individual lives**	Lots of paperwork and folders but the information contained in them is either irrelevant or doesn't get implemented in everyday practice.
Care does not meet the priorities or needs of people living with dementia. People show high levels of distress behaviour or disengagement.	**Personal perspective**	Emotional and physical burnout. High identification of distress but no ability to help effectively.
Poor communication and lack of dementia-aware interpersonal skills by staff. Emphasis on safety and physical appearance.	**Social and psychological support**	Slavish following of techniques. Frequent changes in direction as latest techniques are tried and discarded.

Valuing

Too little emphasis on this element

The first element (V) is about valuing people with dementia in all that we do. In Chapter 3 we recognised that people living with dementia and their families and friends are in danger of not getting equal access to good-quality care. Historically, when there were far fewer people with dementia, services for people with dementia were seen as specialist provision. When Kitwood was first writing, this was indeed the case. Now, every provider of health and social care services for adults needs to recognise that people with dementia and their families are part of core business. So, whether the service is a GP practice, a hospital, a care home or a home-care provider, people with dementia and their families will be core users.

Yet many of these services still do not see themselves as dementia care service providers. The danger in not making it explicit that services are there to be inclusive of all, means that people with significant cognitive impairments will have greater difficulty accessing these services and they are unlikely to meet people's needs. In the worst cases, people living with dementia are seen as the cause of the problem with resources (e.g. referred to as 'bed-blockers') rather than as the victims of a service that is not geared to meet their needs. Valuing people with dementia is something that care providers have to be actively signed up to if they are to implement person-centred care. Staff on the front line may be doing their best but without value being put on the lives of people living with dementia they will be fighting a difficult daily battle and quality will be difficult to sustain.

Only emphasising this element

On the other hand, if person-centred care is seen only as a value base, then it can quickly become a group of empty words or evangelism without a practical application and a body of knowledge. There are some people who can extrapolate practice very easily from a value base, but many others need the implications to be spelt out in rather more concrete terms. The situation can occur where the glossy brochures produced by care providers are full of fine words and promises of valued lives. However, if the 'business' is not really geared up to deliver these promises then these valuing statements become empty words and person-centred care cannot occur.

Influencing change at the valuing level

All of the indicators in the V element will bring about a provider organisation that can deliver and sustain person-centred dementia care. Real transformation occurs when leaders at the top of the organisation are clear in their purpose and outcomes. What they say in the glossy brochure gets translated into what they do in practice, and problems in that translation are identified and solved. The organisation's strategic plan designs a road map for how this is achieved. The idea is followed through to ensure delivery. Key lines of communication, strong alliances and relationships through the different levels of organisational influence are necessary to build change. Having staff roles and job plans that are aligned to the dementia care strategy within the organisation are often the vehicle for implementing change into practice.

Individual lives

Too little emphasis on this element

The second element (I) is the focus on the individual's life. We learnt in Chapter 4 the difficulties that people living with dementia face in holding on to their sense of identity and how this impacts on personhood. Particularly, as dementia progresses and complex individual needs are not assessed and catered for, the provision of person-centred care becomes too chaotic to be deliverable. All of the indicators within the I element require processes and structures to be in place so that staff can 'know' the people they are to care for quickly and easily. If it is nobody's job role to put these processes in place and to supervise their use, care is done on a trial-and-error basis. Sometimes it will be okay, others not.

Only emphasising this element

If person-centred care is just taken to mean individualised care without the other elements of the definition, care can quickly deteriorate into serving needs within a very narrow frame that makes very little difference to the lived experience of dementia. It is possible to do individualised assessments and care without considering the viewpoint of the person with dementia at all. In these cases, the assessment would generally focus on constructs entirely determined by the professional perspective. All service users may have individual care plans that are different from each other but may not prioritise the things that are important for each individual in any way.

This element can get overemphasised in organisations that have appointed a dementia lead who develops lots of assessment forms and processes without really thinking through how these will impact on practice. There can be a danger that the checklist of protocol becomes an end in itself rather than being about the delivery of person-centred care. 'I've got 12 more life stories to complete my target this week,' may not lead to anyone's sense of personhood being maintained! If this is all that person-centred care is taken to mean then a lot of information is generated that never makes a difference to people's lives. Filing cabinets in care facilities around the world are full of information about people's lives but still care staff will not know even the rudimentary facts.

Influencing change at the individual lives level

Many staff and professionals who are employed at the 'dementia-lead' level where they can focus on developing processes involved in the I indicators are in a very strong position to influence the provision of person-centred care. They are often in a position to communicate well with the top decision-makers within an organisation and also to influence directly front-line delivery. They need to develop ways of communicating with those involved in different parts of the organisation to translate person-centred practice into their reality. They need to be able to communicate with those above them to ensure they see person-centred practice as meeting the business objectives. They might be able to see things within the organisation that need to change within the V indicators, such as management ethos or staff training, and they need to be able to form alliances with those above them to help them move forwards.

They also need to be able to work with front-line staff to ensure they have the skills and resources to implement person-centred practice on the front line and to discover where practical barriers might exist. For every new form, process or record it is important to walk this through in an organisation to ensure that it will really benefit people living with dementia. Pilot projects, Plan, Do, Study, Act cycles and reflective practice are the modus operandi of people working at this level to bring about change.

Perspective

Too little emphasis on this element

The third element (P) is about taking the perspective of the person with dementia as the starting point. When staff do not make a serious attempt to think about care from the perspective of the person they are caring for then care becomes trial and error. The level of distress behaviour, or so-called 'challenging behaviour', is likely to be high as people living with dementia struggle to make themselves heard.

Alternatively, people living long-term in care environments with little understanding of their needs may become burnt out in their attempts to communicate needs, and a situation of learnt helplessness and apathy develops. The person with dementia becomes more and more disengaged from the world.

Only emphasising this element

Frequently we come across care situations where there has been an investment in helping front-line health and care staff to become much more aware of the emotional needs of the people with dementia they are supporting, but the skills or resources to help them with those needs have not been addressed or the processes to deliver valuing individualised care have not been developed. This can be the case in organisations that have done lots of 'awareness' training but little else. This puts front-line staff in a position where they are exposed to strong feelings of guilt and helplessness, which over time leads to emotional burnout and disengagement.

Influencing change at the perspectives level

Having a strong empathy with the emotional needs and perspectives of people living with dementia is a strong driver for change. This motivation can be used to work with people in staff teams to improve an individual's quality of life. Maybe there is a person who has unusual or distressing behaviour. Finding out as much a possible about that person's background and health may help shed light on why someone is struggling. Getting help from specialist community health teams may help improve that person's quality of life and may also improve the skills more generally within the team. Suggesting changes in the care environment or in general procedures to those in a position to influence may help. Suggesting a pilot project as a way of bringing about change may be more acceptable than a big change. Publicising successes may inspire more widespread changes.

Supportive social psychology

Too little emphasis on this element

The fourth element (S) is the positive social environment. If care workers, family members and organisations do not have the skills and competencies to provide a positive social environment for people with dementia, then confusion and distress will reign. In providing person-centred care, a supportive and nurturing social environment is the key to maintaining personhood on a day-to-day basis. As the sense of self breaks down, it becomes increasingly important that the relationships that the person with dementia experiences remains strong. As verbal abilities are lost, the importance of warm, accepting human contact through non-verbal channels becomes even more important. When this is absent, the organisation is likely to have an over-reliance on care practices that promote safety and on the aesthetics of the physical care environment. If this is a care home or hospital, it may look good to visitors initially, but the experience of spending time there, particularly for people living with dementia, will be one that is toxic.

Only emphasising this element

There are many care staff and professionals worldwide who instinctively know how to provide care and support that nurtures a sense of well-being and personhood. Delivering compassionate care is a strong driver for many who work in care. There are many others who can learn how to do this by working alongside staff who provide a sense of warmth, inclusivity and empowerment in their everyday interactions. Where there is a strong supportive social psychology that is not backed up by the other elements, however, it is unlikely that this will sustain over time. It will be dependent on individual staff.

If these staff are not appreciated for their skills or their good ideas are not listened to, the chances are that they will move on to another care provider who will value them. Sometimes the delivery of compassionate care gets overlooked. In its place we try to find a new 'quick fix' or technique to put in its place. Person-centred care is about people, not tools and techniques. Without a strong value base, the reason for using these tools in the first place becomes obscured and a slavish following of technique can occur.

Influencing change at the supportive social psychology level

Having a staff team that is skilled in creating a strong social psychological support for people living with dementia is a tremendous asset. Care organisations need to capitalise on this and build teams with people who have this propensity and skillset. Ensuring that staff who have these skills gain respect and recognition through informal means (recognition on a day-to-day basis) and formal means (promotion, appraisal, awards) will spread good practice.

When person-centred care is lost

Many care organisations provide good care. However, our experience suggests that often, care is held together by a few hardworking staff who deliver good care against the odds, through their own personal commitment and resources, rather than being well supported to do so. If these staff resign, are unwell or are on leave, care can deteriorate very quickly and neglectful practice can go unchallenged. This can escalate to the types of extreme neglectful and abusive practice we have seen in undercover films.

It needs a very strong management culture to turn around a failing care home (or hospital) and nurture the culture to remain positive. There is no 'quick fix'. The VIPS indicators and the attention to care culture set out within this book can take years to be firmly established and continual work to retain. The most effective way of promoting health and well-being of people living with dementia in care homes and hospitals is to recruit and retain good-quality staff and leaders of staff. It is they who will be responsible for setting the care culture, as a head teacher is in a school. In order to run a care home or hospital, the board, its senior managers, its facilities managers and its shift leaders must all know what good care looks like and how to manage teams to deliver good-quality care.

Summary

Dementia is a serious problem for all who are affected by it. However, it may be that by taking a more person-centred approach to our care we can avoid some of the suffering that is caused by an absence of care that maintains personhood. This VIPS Framework does not apply just to services for people living with dementia, but it also applies to all who find themselves in a state of dependence and vulnerability. In other words, it applies to every single one of us.

Part 2
The VIPS Framework

The VIPS Framework: Person-centred Care for People Living with Dementia

Using the VIPS Framework

The VIPS definition of person-centred care encompasses four major elements.

V A value base that asserts the absolute value of all human lives regardless of age or cognitive ability.

I An individualised approach, recognising uniqueness.

P Understanding the world from the perspective of the person identified as needing support.

S Providing a social environment that supports psychological needs.

These elements have been described in great detail in Part 1 of this book. In Part 2 the VIPS Framework Tool is presented.

This tool is designed to help providers of health and care services for people living with dementia to assess the relative strengths and weaknesses with regard to providing person-centred care. It details six key indicators under each element that demonstrate person-centred care. There is an additional indicator under the S element about the importance of relationships. For each indicator, you are asked to reflect on how your organisation is performing. You can then use this to derive an action plan for service quality improvements.

There are a number of different ways you can use this framework. We have found that a good starting place is to complete the document as a group, preferably using people who have different roles within your organisation and with input from people who use your service. It is unlikely that one person will be able to answer it all. Indeed, it is the different perspectives on particular indicators that can often highlight an area of service improvement.

We use the term 'care providers' in the broadest sense. It covers all those providing a service for people living with dementia in their own homes, day care, housing schemes, care homes or health and hospital care.

We encourage you also to utilise the Care Fit for VIPS website. This is a free website www.carefitforvips.co.uk, although you will need to register to get full functionality. The original version was specifically aimed at staff working in care homes but now versions are also available for domiciliary care, day care and housing. It is also widely used by hospital and health staff. Each version uses the same 25 indicators but how these indicators are described in practical terms varies between the different types of service provision.

The website has pages on each indicator where the provider is asked a series of questions to assess their performance on each one. These questions and reflection points are similar to those in this book. When indicators are rated more highly, the colour on the website changes for that indicator. For the paper version produced here we have created reflection points that should be applicable to a wide range of health and care providers, although different providers may have a different emphasis or scope regarding certain indicators.

On the website there are also pages that provide a Plan, Do, Study, Act action-planning cycle for any area that requires a quality improvement plan. In order to assist with quality improvements there is an extensive collection of web links to books, articles, training resources and YouTube clips for each indicator. These are updated as new resources are identified. All resources are vetted to make sure they are of reasonable quality and person-centred.

The title of each indicator is provided below.

Valuing indicators

V1	**Vision**: Does everyone know what we stand for and share the vision?
V2	**Human resources**: Are systems in place to ensure staff know that they are valued as a precious resource?
V3	**Management ethos**: Are management practices empowering to staff delivering direct care to ensure care is person-centred?
V4	**Training and practice development**: Are there systems in place to support the development of a workforce skilled in person-centred dementia care? Do staff know that supporting people living with dementia is treated as skilled and important work?
V5	**The service environments**: Are there supportive and inclusive physical and social environments for people living with cognitive disability? Do our places help people?
V6	**Quality assurance**: Are Continuous Quality Improvement mechanisms in place that are driven by knowing and acting upon needs and concerns of people with dementia and their supporters? Do we strive to get better all the time?

Individual lives indicators

I1	**Individual support and care**: Do our care and support plans promote individual identity showing that everyone is unique, with hopes, fears, strengths and needs?
I2	**Regular reviews**: Do we recognise and respond to change?
I3	**Personal possessions**: Do people have their favourite and important things around them? Do we know why they're meaningful for them?
I4	**Individual preferences**: Are a person's likes and dislikes, preferences and choices listened to, known about and acted upon?
I5	**Life stories**: Are a person's important relationships, significant life stories and key events known about and referenced in everyday activities?
I6	**Activity and occupation**: Is a person's day full of purpose and engagement with the world regardless of their needs and abilities?

Personal perspective indicators

P1	**Communication is key**: Are we alert to all the ways that people living with dementia communicate and are we skilled at responding appropriately?
P2	**Empathy and acceptable risk**: Do we put ourselves in the position of the person we're supporting and think about the world from their point of view?
P3	**Physical environment**: Is this a place that helps someone living with dementia to feel comfortable, safe and at ease?
P4	**Physical health needs**: Are we alert to, responsive to and optimising people's health and well-being?
P5	**Challenging behaviour as communication**: Do we always consider and act on what a person is trying to tell us though their behavioural communication? Do we look for underlying reasons rather than seeking to 'manage' it?
P6	**Advocacy**: Do we speak out on behalf of people living with dementia to make sure their rights, respect and dignity are upheld?

Socially supportive environment indicators

S1	**Inclusion**: Are people helped to feel part of what is going on around them and supported to participate in a way that they are able?
S2	**Respect**: Does the support we provide show people that they are respected as individuals with unique identities, strengths and needs?
S3	**Warmth**: Does the atmosphere we create help people to feel welcomed, wanted and accepted?
S4	**Validation**: Are people's emotions and feelings recognised, taken seriously and responded to?
S5	**Enabling**: Does the support we provide help people to be as active and involved in their lives as possible? Are people treated as partners in their care?
S6	**Part of the community**: Does our service do all it can to keep people connected with their local community and the local community connected with the service?
S7	**Relationships**: Do we know about, welcome and involve the people who are important to a person?

Within Part 2 of this book, care providers are asked to reflect on how well they think they are doing for each indicator on the following scale:

- **Excellent**: This is where the provider has no doubt they are reaching the highest standards within the indicator, they have maintained this over a period of time and it is consistent across their whole service.

- **Good**: This is where the provider is sure they have achieved a high standard against the indicator, but they have some concerns about the consistency or sustainability of the standard in some areas of their service.

- **Okay**: This is an adequate performance that means they can provide evidence of the indicator being met most of the time, or they have elements of good practice that could be introduced more widely across the organisation.

- **Needs more work**: This is where the provider does not know how they are doing on a particular indicator, where they are concerned that they have not addressed it or where they need to identify the building blocks to its being met on a consistent basis.

The VIPS Framework can be used on at least three different levels:

1. **Raising awareness of person-centred care across the organisation**: Using it in this way, a group leader uses the questions to facilitate a discussion about each question. The composition of the group will depend on the size of the care organisation and the main aim in bringing people together. This could be a naturally occurring team such as a ward team, a home-care team or the executive board of a care provider. It is probably most useful, however, to have a group of around 10–12 people who work at different levels within the organisation or who have responsibility for different areas. Depending on the type of service and the openness of the organisation, the discussion will be enriched further by having people who use the service, or who support people using the service, to be part of this discussion. Different group members might want to fill in the questionnaire online before coming together to share results.

The discussion will generate many things in its own right. There will be areas to celebrate where the organisation recognises things that it already does well and it may want to publicise these further. There will be other areas where there is a mismatch of experience between different group members.

Sometimes this occurs in the difference between what is meant to happen according to policies and procedures and what is actually happening in reality. There may be variation across the organisation, suggesting that effective practice needs to be shared. There will be other areas where the group identifies gaps in provision and may generate an initial discussion of how this could be addressed. This sort of group facilitation needs skilful handling to ensure participants are comfortable in sharing information and in challenging each other's assumptions.

2. **Evidence collection and benchmarking**: This would be a more formal means of using the framework to check how practice measures up in reality. Most organisations think they are doing better than they actually are! Ways of evidencing could include reviewing paperwork and records, interviewing staff and service users, focus groups on particular topics, questionnaires, observations of practice and monitoring key indicators and critical incidents. This sort of evidence collection and analysis requires skills in evaluation and audit, and it is important to remember that there is little substitute for spending time in a service talking to those who experience care and support and those who deliver it on the front line.

3. **Action planning for improvements in key elements**: It may be that an organisation needs to focus on one or two areas to really make an impact on practice. This might be in terms of particular working groups or learning sets coming together on specific elements or indicators. The indicators can be used to identify the key areas of concern. Using the indicators in this way requires skills in project management and practice development.

Person-centred care requires sign-up to working in this way across the whole care-provider organisation if it is to be sustained over any length of time. Particular elements require leadership at different levels:

- The first element – **valuing people** – requires leadership from those responsible for leading the organisation at a senior level.

- The second element – **individualised care** – requires leadership particularly from those responsible for setting care standards and procedures within the care organisation.

- The final two elements – **personal perspectives** and **supportive social environment** – require leadership from those responsible for the day-to-day management and provision of care.

As we have emphasised throughout Part 1 of this book, when evaluating your service or thinking about areas of change and improvement it is important to consider how the overall culture of an organisation will help or hinder what can happen on the ground. It is really important than when you evaluate how well you are doing, or prioritise the areas that you want to work on, you consider the impact of the organisational culture on what you are trying to achieve. Here, we have reproduced the key messages regarding positive care cultures for people living with dementia and complex needs as established from the CHOICE project.

> We all **work together** to deliver the best care. **We all matter** to each other. We **empower and support front-line staff** to empower and support people living with dementia. Our leadership **protects front-line service delivery** as paramount. On a day-to day basis this means that every day is different and staff **constantly look to make things better** for the people they care for. We help people to **enjoy places where they spend time** and to be **active in a way that fulfils them every day.**

The VIPS Framework reflection points and evidence

Name of care provider: ....

Date: ....

Type of organisation: ....

People contributing to rating our performance: ....

....

....

....

....

....

....

....

....

....

....

....

....

....

....

....

....

....

....

....

....

....

....

....

....

✓

Valuing

Valuing people with dementia and those who care for them: promoting citizenship rights and entitlements regardless of age or cognitive impairment and rooting out discriminatory practice.

V1 Vision: Does everyone know what we stand for and share the vision?	How are we doing?
Reflection points: Valuing people begins at the top. The vision states your organisation's priorities and aims and implies the values that are the centre of the work you do. It takes hard work towards a clear and consistent goal to make progress and maintain standards. You need to consider how different aspects of your organisation's culture impact on achieving the vision in practice. By clearly communicating a commitment to person-centred practice you enable everyone to know what their priorities should be and create a standard by which you can be held to account. **Consider these statements:** • There is a vision (or mission) statement that makes person-centred care a priority. • Our vision statement is easy for all staff, people living with dementia and their families and friends to understand. It avoids jargon, uses simple words, phrases and pictures and is available in different formats. • Our vision statement helps everyone judge how well we are doing in achieving our aims in practice. • People living with dementia and their family, friends and staff can contribute to forming the vision statement. • All staff know the essence of what our vision is and what they can do to put it into practice when supporting people on a day-to-day basis. • The board (or those who govern the organisation) use the vision statement to guide their decisions and it is referred to when changes are made to the service. **This can be evidenced by**: • an audit of materials available to service users about the service • talking to staff or staff surveys • observing what is experienced by people receiving support • talking to or surveying people who use and visit the service • examining admissions or new service-user pathways.	Excellent Good Okay Needs more work

✓

V2 Human resources: Are systems in place to ensure staff know that they are valued as a precious resource?	How are we doing?
Reflection points: Running any service that provides care and support for people has to be a people business. Staff will only be able to show that they value the people they care for if they themselves feel valued. They need to be supported by their organisation to do their jobs. You need to consider how well the different aspects of your organisation's culture impact on the daily emotional and practical support that staff receive. If an organisation listens and responds to their staff needs, staff are free to listen and respond to the individuals they support. This is something that should inform an organisation's approach to recruitment, formal supervision, staff training and development as well as day-today interactions and informal support of staff. **Consider these statements**: • Our recruitment procedures focus on getting the right people for our services and the people we support. • A system of staff supervision and appraisal is fully implemented and informal day-to-day mechanisms for support are in place. • Staff are encouraged to work as a team, with systems (such as handovers, shift rotas etc.) encouraging this. • The stresses and difficulties experienced by front-line staff are recognised, and staff are supported to talk about them and deal with them appropriately. • Staff can identify what action they would take if they were worried about a person's support or could see an opportunity to improve things. They feel confident and supported to express their feelings and ideas. • Staff are encouraged to develop their skills and have a career pathway. **This can be evidenced by**: • staff surveys, interviews and discussions • staff portfolios of impact on service design and delivery • audits of recruitment and supervision procedures • external accreditation, such as Investors in People.	Excellent Good Okay Needs more work

V3 Management ethos: Are management practices empowering to staff delivering direct care to ensure care is person-centred?	How are we doing?
Reflection points: Good support and care need good staff; good staff need good management. To support someone in a person-centred way, staff need to be able to draw on their own emotional and physical resources. To do this well, staff need an environment that values their work and helps them to deal with demands of the job. You need to consider how your organisation's culture facilitates or obstructs staff ability to be empowered to act on behalf of people they support on a day-to-day basis. Structure, systems and routine are essential, but they must be fair and flexible. An open, can-do culture means staff can grow into the job, getting better and better at what they do. **Consider these statements**: • There is a culture of reviewing and aiming to improve what we do in our service. Staff and people using and visiting the service are involved. • Staff frequently come to senior staff and management with questions, ideas and challenges for how to improve the service, and these are acted upon. • There is good communication across all teams and shifts, allowing sufficient time to share information, discuss concerns and problem-solve together. • The service is viewed by all as a community to which all belong, rather than a 'them-and-us' approach. • Staff feel that the work they do is important and that they can make positive differences to people's lives. • Staff are supported to reflect on their own practice and identify strengths and weakness. Staff feel they can talk about difficulties and will receive support and encouragement. **This can be evidenced by**: • surveys, interviews and discussions with staff • records of staff meetings, supervisions and procedures • collection and analysis of comments, compliments and complaints • observing the day-to-day experiences of staff.	Excellent Good Okay Needs more work

V4 Training and staff development: Are there systems in place to support the development of a workforce skilled in person-centred dementia care? Do staff know that supporting people living with dementia is treated as skilled and important work?	How are we doing?
Reflection points: Supporting a person with dementia is a skilled task. Maintaining person-centred care for people with dementia is not easy. Caring well for people is emotionally and physically intense. Staff need strong values, self-awareness and a good understanding of dementia, along with specific skills such as communication and risk-taking. These should develop continually as they reflect on their work through training, supervision and team sessions. You need to consider whether your organisation's culture enables staff to reflect and adapt on a daily basis to the challenges of their work. **Consider these statements**: • Our staff induction ensures everyone is positive about working with people with dementia. Negative attitudes, language and practices are constructively challenged whenever they occur. • Our organisation has a clear strategy and resources to train and develop staff for the benefit of people who receive support. • Everyone is supported to reflect on their practice through supervision, mentoring and day-to-day support and to develop and share their expertise. • Dementia care is recognised as a specialist skill and our staff are trained and supported accordingly. • The practices and systems we use on a daily basis enable staff to put their training into practice. • We have ways that we support visitors, family and friends to develop and contribute to their own caring role. **This can be evidenced by**: • surveys, interviews and discussions with staff • records of training and continued action learning initiatives • analysis of staff skills and development needs • critical incident analysis and notes of reflective practice meetings.	Excellent Good Okay Needs more work

V5 Service environments: Are there supportive and inclusive physical and social environments for people living with cognitive disability? Do our places help people?	How are we doing?
Reflection points: We would expect a service to be designed, or adapted, so that it is accessible by someone who uses a wheelchair or someone who has a visual impairment. When we aim to provide care for people with dementia, we should ensure that our building and social environment are suitable for them and actively support their physical and emotional well-being. You should think about how well your organisation's culture helps staff to adapt on a daily basis to people's needs. **Consider these statements**: • The use of layout, decoration and facilities in the service are designed to encourage independence, help people to feel safe and secure and make it easy for them to access help when they need it. • The use of layout and decoration in the service are designed to help people get around and feel familiarity, despite the challenges they face (whether through confusion, memory loss or physical or sensory difficulties). • People can spend time in a pleasant and safe outside space whenever they wish. • The layout and facilities are used in a way that allows people privacy and familiarity but also enables social contact in pairs or groups of different size. • Visitors, family and friends are welcomed, helped and encouraged to be part of people's daily lives. • All staff who may come into contact with someone with dementia have the communication skills necessary to engage appropriately, put them at ease and respond to their needs. **This can be evidenced by**: • audits of physical environments • discussions, interviews and surveys of people who use services, visitors and families/friends • observations of staff practice • observations of the daily experiences of people receiving support • training records and skills analysis • records of activity and occupation for people receiving support.	Excellent Good Okay Needs more work

V6 Quality assurance: Are Continuous Quality Improvement mechanisms in place that are driven by knowing and acting upon needs and concerns of people with dementia and their supporters? Do we strive to get better all the time?	How are we doing?
Reflection points: Unless we make a conscious effort to find out what life is like for people who receive support or work in or visit our service we can fail to see what needs to be improved. Seeking the opinions and experiences of people who receive support from our service is crucial to identifying what might need to change. We should think about the way in which our overall organisation's culture affects staff's ability to receive and act on requests and ideas for improvement. A complaints procedure is a good beginning, but we need to positively seek out comments, issues and problems on a daily basis to create an open culture. **Consider these statements**: • We have ways of finding out how safe, engaged and happy people feel with their support. These include regular, formal approaches but also capture day-to-day and ad-hoc opportunities for feedback. • We positively encourage feedback from external visitors to the service, whether family and friends or professionals. • Senior staff make themselves available to respond to daily issues and concerns. People receiving support and visitors feel confident in their ability to solve problems. • All our staff feel they have a role in making people happy, involved and safe. They feel confident and supported to raise concerns about poor practice, and they are encouraged to do so. • We have a compliments, comments and complaints procedure that everyone understands and has the necessary support to use. • We have ways of capturing the experiences of people who may not be able to communicate worries themselves.	Excellent Good Okay Needs more work

This can be evidenced by:

- discussions, interviews and surveys of people who receive support
- observations of the daily experiences of people receiving support, particularly the most vulnerable
- records/audits of meetings and supervisions
- results of formal quality-assurance processes
- external quality-assurance accreditation.

Points for action	Overall performance on valuing

✓

Individual lives

Recognising that all people are different with a unique history and personality, physical and psychological strengths and needs, and social and economic resources that will affect their response to dementia.

I1 Care and support planning: Do our care and support plans promote individual identity showing that everyone is unique, with hopes, fears, strengths and needs?	How are we doing?
Reflection points: We are all unique, with different talents, hopes, fears, strengths and weaknesses. A person with dementia is no different, so care that we provide must be a based on an understanding of the person as an individual. It takes time and effort to get to know someone well and what is important for one person may not suit the next. We need to consider how well our organisational culture affects the flexibility and responsiveness of the support we provide. Knowing a person well can help us to provide good support, solve problems more easily and involve people fully in their own lives.	
Consider these statements: • We gather as much information as possible about a person's life history before they receive our support and continue to do so on an ongoing basis. • Each person's plan for care and support identifies what they can do and what their strengths and wishes are, as well as identifying what support they may need. • We recognise people's emotional and spiritual needs, including dreams and goals, as well as their physical needs. • Our plans for care tell us what support each person needs to be as independent as possible and involved in daily decisions. • We regularly update and review our plans for care to make sure new things we find out about a person are recognised. • We use lots of different sources to help us develop our plans for care: the people themselves, their family and friends, observations of the people, staff working with them and any specialist advice.	Excellent Good Okay Needs more work
This can be evidenced by: • discussions, interviews and surveys with people who receive support and their family and visitors • observations of care and support practice and experiences • audits of care plans and their implementation • individual care pathways and case tracking.	

✓

I2 Regular reviews: Do we recognise and respond to change?	How are we doing?
Reflection points: Throughout our lives, our needs, abilities and interests change. For someone with dementia this is just as true, and the support they need may change from day to day or hour to hour. To provide good, person-centred care we must be able to notice and respond quickly to these changes. You need to think about how well your organisation's culture impacts on front-line support delivery and its ability to recognise and adapt to necessary changes. **Consider these statements**: • There are regular, formal reviews of people's support, but daily changes are noticed and responded to. • Staff work flexibly so that changes in a person can be easily recognised and responded to each day. • All staff have easy access to information about a person's support plan so that they can use it in their work and notice any changes quickly. • Our plans for care are living documents that everyone can contribute to on an ongoing basis: individuals themselves, their family and visitors and staff. • Staff know when to seek advice from others (inside or outside the service itself) so that they can understand and respond to changes. • We have links to other services (such as community mental health teams or specialist services) that can help us understand and respond to changes that we see. **This can be evidenced by**: • discussions, interviews and surveys of people receiving support and their family and visitors • observations of practice, support experiences and daily routines • audits of care and support plans and assessments • care pathways and case tracking • records of communication from people and their families and visitors and professionals.	Excellent Good Okay Needs more work

I3 Personal possessions: Do people have their favourite and important things around them? Do we know why they're meaningful for them?	How are we doing?
Reflection points: We all have favourite belongings that are important to us because they trigger memories and feelings about significant events or people in our lives. What might be of great value to us may appear meaningless to someone else. Textures, smells or sounds may evoke particular experiences or events in our lives and help us to feel comfort and familiarity even in a strange or new situation. You need to consider how well your organisation's culture enables these possessions and experiences to be used with people on a daily basis. Person-centred care means finding out about and using these important possessions when we're supporting a person. **Consider these statements**: • People are encouraged to personalise their spaces with their possessions, furniture, photos etc. • People have their own clothes and choices about them each day, (the type, style and material are what the person is used to or wants). • Staff respect and take care of an individual's personal possessions. • Staff can be seen to use personal possessions to engage and interact with a person. • Staff encourage the use of personal possessions by an individual, particularly when someone may not be able to ask for them or access them by themselves. • When new items are needed, the person is involved in their selection and attention is paid to what might be familiar for the person. **This can be evidenced by**: • discussions, interviews and surveys of people receiving support and their family and visitors • observations of practice and staff use of possessions • physical environment audits • audits of care and support plans and assessments.	Excellent Good Okay Needs more work

✓

I4 Individual preferences: Are a person's likes, dislikes, preferences and choices listened to, known about and acted upon?	How are we doing?
Reflection points: It is easy to take for granted the small choices we all make every day. Simple, everyday decisions such as what time to get up, whether to have a hot or cold drink and where to walk or sit seem unimportant until we imagine what life would be like if others controlled these events. Many people with dementia will rely on other people to encourage, listen to and act on their preferences. You need to consider how well your organisation's culture enables these preferences to be found out and acted on. When a person is involved and in control of their daily lives, it will improve their well-being enormously. Person-centred care means finding out about individuals' likes, dislikes and preferences and acting on them every day. **Consider these statements**: • A person's likes, dislikes, routines and preferences are established through communicating with them and their family and friends. Any changes are recognised and communicated to staff and family and friends. • A person's likes and dislikes in all aspects of their lives are part of their support plan and are acted upon by staff every day. • Each individual has a different daily routine that corresponds to their own preferences. • Any regular event (such as a mealtime) is flexibly managed to accommodate individual preferences, needs and changes. • Staff show an understanding of how to involve people in making decisions, expressing choice and communicating likes and dislikes. • People are allowed to change their mind and staff work flexibly so changes can be responded to. **This can be evidenced by**: • discussions, interviews and surveys with people who receive support • observations of practice and daily routines • audits of care plans and assessments • discussions and interviews with staff.	Excellent Good Okay Needs more work

✓

I5 Life history: Are a person's important relationships, significant life stories and key events known about and referenced in everyday activities?	How are we doing?
Reflection points: It is easy to assess a person on face value and ignore their individual history and experiences. However, it is our life experiences and relationships that make us who we are. Person-centred care requires in-depth knowledge of someone's life history and the key events that bring joy or sadness and an understanding of the people and activities that are or have been important to someone. Without this knowledge, positive and identity-confirming communication and care is very difficult, and a person's behaviour and reactions are very difficult to interpret. You should think about the ways in which your organisation's culture supports the ongoing collection and use of such information	
Consider these statements:	
• Each person who receives support, along with their family and friends, is encouraged and helped to create a life story book, memory box or something similar.	
• Staff show an interest in a person's unique history and use it to communicate and engage with a person.	Excellent
• Staff spend time with individuals talking, looking at photos and sharing memories. When helping people with personal care, staff use this as an opportunity to engage and interact with the person.	Good Okay Needs more work
• Families and friends are encouraged to share anecdotes, memories, photos or possessions that will help staff get to know the person. Staff keep families and friends up to date about the person's life.	
• People have access to music, everyday objects and photos from a time and place of which they have strong memories.	
• Staff use their knowledge of a person's life to interpret behaviour and communication and seek to find out more information when this proves difficult.	
This can be evidenced by:	
• discussions, interviews and surveys with people who receive support and their family, friends and visitors	
• observations of support received by people and of staff practice	
• audits of care plans and assessments	
• reviews of life stories, memory boxes etc.	

✓

I6 Activity and occupation: Is a person's day full of purpose and engagement with the world, regardless of their needs and abilities?	How are we doing?
Reflection points: Our happiest times are often when we are engaged in an activity we enjoy, whether this is fixing a car, painting a picture or having a chat with a friend. Any length of time without meaningful occupation can lead to boredom, frustration and distress, and if this continues over time a person can give up on the world around them. Person-centred care means finding a way for every day to have meaning for each individual and exploring ways to keep a person interested and engaged. You need to think about the ways your organisation's culture helps this to happen every day. A schedule of regular group activities is not enough; spontaneous events, involvement in daily tasks and one-to-one interaction mean that individuals are genuinely occupied. **Consider these statements**: • All staff see activity and occupation as an integral part of their work and take opportunities as and when they arise. • Ordinary daily tasks such as cooking, cleaning, gardening or reading the paper are recognised as opportunities to involve and occupy people. • Staff take the lead of the people themselves and encourage any activity that seems meaningful to an individual. Those who are not able to initiate an activity are supported by staff to do so. • A pleasant and safe outside space is always available and accessible, and it provides a range of sensory experiences. • The physical environment and objects around the person encourage them to be active and occupied. • People are supported to attend local events and to attend activities outside of the home. **This can be evidenced by**: • discussions, interviews and surveys with people receiving support and their family and friends • physical environment audits • records of people's activity and occupation • observations of people's day-to-day experiences • audits of care plans and assessments.	Excellent Good Okay Needs more work

✓

Points for action	Overall performance on individualised care

Personal perspectives

Looking at the world from the perspective of the person with dementia: Recognising that each person's experience has its own psychological validity, that people act from this perspective and that empathy with this perspective has its own therapeutic potential.

P1 Communication is key: Are we alert to all the ways that people living with dementia communicate and are we skilled at responding appropriately?	How are we doing?
Reflection points: Communication is about more than words. It includes behaviour, facial expression and body language. Successful communication requires a two-way interaction; it's not just about a person having something to tell us, but also us being willing and able to listen. We need to think about how our organisation's culture encourages good, continual two-way communication. People living with dementia can find that their preferences and opinions are ignored because they have difficulty communicating. To make person-centred care happen, everyone in the home setting needs to communicate well. **Consider these statements**: • We see staff using many different styles of communication every day. They are responsive to non-verbal communication. • Staff actively demonstrate how to encourage a person's involvement, support each person to make decisions and do not take action without consulting a person. • Staff show awareness of the impact of their non-verbal communication on the people they support. • When decisions might be too complex for people to make themselves, staff know how to encourage involvement, who else to consult and how to ensure the best decision is made. • We know which residents have sight and hearing loss, and we use all the resources available to assist people actively in their communication. • We understand the importance of people hearing and using the language that is their mother tongue. Staff use all the resources available to them to assist people actively in their communication. They are aware of individual cultural issues around communication. **This can be evidenced by**: • observations of people's experiences of support • observations of staff practice • audits of care plans and assessments.	Excellent Good Okay Needs more work

✓

P2 Empathy and acceptable risk: Do we put ourselves in the position of the person we're supporting and think about the world from their point of view?	How are we doing?
Reflection points: It is easy to assume that everyone else experiences the world in the same way that we do and forget that another may see things differently or interpret our approach in a way that we didn't intend. In order to be person-centred, we must try to see the world through a person's eyes. How might a situation feel to them? What is important to them? What are their opinions and priorities in any situation? You need to think about the impact of your organisation's culture on staff's ability to do this every day. Without considering the person's own perspective, there is a risk that we will err on the side of caution and do what is easiest and safest for us, rather than what will increase a person's comfort, occupation and happiness.	
Consider these statements: • We know how each person shows us, moment to moment, if they are happy or unhappy. • Staff show that they think about how their behaviour, approach and communication might make others feel and are able to change it in response. • We regularly try to imagine how an activity or event may be experienced by a person with dementia, and we suggest changes as a result. • If someone is distressed, or behaving in a way that is difficult to deal with, we think first about how that person might be experiencing the world. • Our risk assessments aim to find a way for someone to do something in a safer way, rather than to prevent them doing it at all. • Our plans for care, and the day-to-day lives of people, show that we support people to take risks that could improve their emotional well-being.	Excellent Good Okay Needs more work
This can be evidenced by: • observations of people's experience of support • audits of care plans and assessments • audits of risk assessments • discussions with staff regarding risk • observations of staff practice.	

✓

P3 Physical environment: Is this a place that helps someone living with dementia to feel comfortable, safe and at ease?	How are we doing?
Reflection points: Feeling comfortable, safe and at ease in an environment is important for everyone. For people with dementia it is especially important, as other parts of their dementia may decrease their feelings of familiarity and comfort. Temperature, noise levels, smell, colour and general atmosphere can all enhance someone's feeling of 'home' or worsen anxiety and distress. You need to think about how your organisation's culture may impact on staff's ability to think about this each day. On a day-to-day basis, we may not have control over the fabric of the building but can still play a big part in making the environment comfortable, stimulating and safe. **Consider these statements**: • We understand the importance of people being able to get familiar with new environments, through exploration and helpful signage etc. Staff ensure people are shown where things are repeatedly and assist people whenever they appear unsure. • People are enabled to move around the environment freely and safely. They can easily get help to move around if they need it. • We understand that noise levels and sudden changes in these can be distressing. Staff are vigilant about the impact of background noise. • We understand that temperature levels can feel very different for those receiving support and those working in an environment. Staff are vigilant about changes in temperature and they manage this for the comfort of people receiving support. • We understand that lighting levels are important for enabling people. Staff are vigilant about changes in lighting and the impact throughout the environment. • We regularly think about what the physical environment must be like for people receiving support and improve it when needed. **This can be evidenced by**: • physical environment audits • observations of the experiences of those receiving support • discussions, interviews and surveys with people receiving support and their family and visitors.	Excellent Good Okay Needs more work

P4 Physical health: Are we alert to, responsive to and optimising people's health and well-being?	How are we doing?
Reflection points: Most people will encounter physical health problems from time to time. These can be difficult to identify in a person with dementia, as they may not be able to tell us easily about their symptoms. However, if we don't notice or respond to physical health problems it can mean a person is left untreated or in pain and this will make their confusion worse. This can contribute to behaviour that may be challenging. We need to consider how well our organisation's culture enables staff to notice, respond to and seek external advice regarding these issues when needed. Helping a person to be physically healthy through vigilance, activity, environment and a balanced diet are all part of good care and can reduce the impact of dementia on a person's well-being. **Consider these statements**: • We know the signs of pain for each person we support. • We investigate the possible physical causes of any changes in behaviour, rather than assuming it is related to dementia. • We think about and act on the sensory needs of each person (including their hearing aids, glasses etc.). • We create opportunities for people to choose healthy lifestyles through physical activity and a balanced diet. • We take measures to ensure people's medication is appropriate and is reviewed regularly. • People have the same access to health care services (GP, district nurses, podiatrist, mental health services etc.) as they would if they were living without dementia. **This can be evidenced by**: • records and analysis of hospital, GP etc. visits • audits of pain assessments for each person • audits of sensory need records within care plans • audits of medication and medication reviews • observations of medication administration • observations of experiences of people receiving support, particularly around pain, health and sensory needs.	Excellent Good Okay Needs more work

P5 Challenging behaviour as communication: Do we always consider and act on what a person is trying to tell us though their behavioural communication? Do we look for underlying reasons rather than seeking to 'manage' it?	How are we doing?
Reflection points: Behaviour is a form of communication. There is always a reason for the way a person behaves, although it may not always be obvious and it is very easy to jump to conclusions or seek a 'quick fix' solution. Person-centred care means trying to understand what someone is telling us through their behaviour: what may have made them feel a certain way and how to see the world from their point of view. You need to think about how your organisation's culture impacts on staff's ability to respond appropriately to these sorts of issues. **Consider these statements:** • We understand that people living with dementia have difficulty communicating in a straightforward way. All staff try to understand what it is that someone is trying to communicate through their behaviours. • We try to look for the triggers and reasons why a person might act in a certain way. • We try to create a physical and social environment that avoids those triggers for each person. • We speak to people's family and friends to try and uncover reasons for behaviours and work out solutions. • Staff are supported to respond to behaviours in an appropriate way and are encouraged to talk about the impact it may have on them and other staff. • Medication is used only as a last resort when there is evidence that it might help. Anti-psychotic medication is used only as a last resort or when there is evidence that it will help. Regular reviews are in place for people on this type of medication. **This can be evidenced by**: • discussions, interviews or surveys with staff • audits and analysis of prescriptions and medication administration • records of critical incident or reflective meetings • observations of practice.	Excellent Good Okay Needs more work

P6 Advocacy: Do we speak out on behalf of people living with dementia to make sure their rights, respect and dignity are upheld?	How are we doing?
Reflection points: Everyone is entitled to basic human rights: to be treated fairly, with respect and dignity and to live free from abuse. It is easy to take them for granted when we can speak out for ourselves and make sure that we are listened to. However, people with dementia may not be able to speak out themselves or may be ignored by others. It is the duty of those supporting and caring for them to ensure that their rights are protected. You need to think about the ways in which your organisation's culture promotes an understanding of these rights. Person-centred care, based on knowledge of a person's history, preferences and ways of communicating will help protect those rights. **Consider these statements**: • We help people to get independent advocacy if they have no one independent to speak up on their behalf. • Everyone who lives here is seen as equal. Any singling out or scapegoating of individuals is challenged immediately and not tolerated. • When situations arise that cause distress or conflict, staff, the person, their family/friends and outside expertise are involved to find solutions. • Staff apply the principles of the Mental Capacity Act (or relevant government policy) in their daily practice. • Staff are encouraged to discuss the difficulties of meeting individuals' rights and also managing competing interests. • Staff have training on rights, dignity, respect and preventing abuse and neglect. The service's systems help them to apply this on a daily basis. **This can be evidenced by**: • individual case tracking and audits of individual care pathways • discussions, interviews and surveys of people receiving support and their family and visitors • records of critical incident or reflective meetings • training records.	Excellent Good Okay Needs more work

✓

Points for action	Overall performance on service-user perspective

✓

Social environment

Providing a supportive social environment: recognising that all human life is grounded in relationships, and that people living with dementia need an enriched social environment that both compensates for their impairment and fosters opportunities for personal growth.

S1 Inclusion: Are people helped to feel part of what is going on around them and supported to participate in a way that they are able?	How are we doing?
Reflection points: Everyone needs to feel part of what is going on around them. We like to be included in activities and conversations, especially if they are about us. It is easy for people with dementia to be ignored or excluded from their daily lives, even by well-meaning people. Conversations can take place over someone's head, assumptions can be made about what a person wants and care can be done to a person rather than with their involvement. We need to think about how our organisation's culture helps staff to think about this on a daily basis. Person-centred care keeps the person at the forefront of everything we do or say and helps people show their preferences and feelings. **Consider these statements**: • All staff recognise the importance of making someone feel included and demonstrate this in their interactions. • We always involve people in discussions or tasks that relate to them, even if we are unsure they can give an opinion or input. • We never talk about someone in front of them without them being part of the conversation. Staff do not talk about people in front of others. • Staff can be seen to try different types of communication with different people to engage them as much as possible. • When tasks need to be carried out, a person is told what is happening, communicated with throughout and encouraged to be involved. • Our plans for care include information on how best to involve a person and how they might indicate a choice or preference. **This can be evidenced by**: • observations of people's experiences • discussions, interviews and surveys with people receiving support and their family and friends.	Excellent Good Okay Needs more work

S2 Respect: Does the support we provide show people that they are respected as individuals with unique identities, strengths and needs?	How are we doing?
Reflection points: When people show us respect it tells us that they value us as an individual and accept that our beliefs, experiences and opinions are important. We need to recognise the wealth of life experience that a person has, which often means they know the world and their own needs better than we do. We need to think about how our organisation's culture impacts upon staff's ability to demonstrate this respect through their practice. Person-centred care means that we need to accept that each person we care for will have strengths, weaknesses and idiosyncrasies just like anyone else. **Consider these statements**: • Staff know each person's life story and use it positively in their daily interactions. • We do not expect people to change their behaviours or preferences to fit in with the service we provide. Service provision is adapted to meet the needs of people. • Staff understand what dignity means and they can show how they maintain it on a daily basis. • We understand that we often know very private information about people, so we are careful about when and where we talk about it. • Staff do not ridicule, tell off or patronise people. If this happens it is challenged immediately by those around them. • The language we use to talk about people is respectful and it avoids labels and judgemental words. **This can be evidenced by**: • observations of people's experiences • discussions, interviews and surveys with people receiving support and their family, friends and visitors • discussions, interviews and surveys with staff • audits of care plans and daily records with regard to language use.	Excellent Good Okay Needs more work

✓

S3 Warmth: Does the atmosphere we create help people to feel welcomed, wanted and accepted?	How are we doing?
Reflection points: Feeling loved and cared for is vital if we are to feel able to manage the day-to-day challenges of life. If we feel welcomed and wanted by those around us and are met with genuine concern, smiles and helpfulness, we feel comfortable, confident and relaxed. If people with dementia do not experience this they can be left feeling frightened, angry, frustrated, depressed or withdrawn. This can also lead to communicating those feelings through behaviour. You need to think about how our organisation's culture impacts upon staff's ability to create an atmosphere of warmth. Person-centred care means creating a warm atmosphere, and this comes from the daily interactions between everyone in the home. **Consider these statements**: • Staff demonstrate an understanding of the impact of their own behaviour and verbal/non-verbal communication on the people they support. • We can consistently see non-verbal communication from each resident that indicates comfort and relaxation. • Staff respond quickly when someone's communication appears to suggest unhappiness or distress. • We understand that people may become withdrawn. Staff offer warm and gentle encouragement to residents who find it difficult to reach out. • Families, friends and visitors are welcomed and made to feel valued and important to the care of their loved one. • Confrontation is avoided at all times. When there are disagreements or difficulties, these are dealt with professionally and away from people receiving support. **This can be evidenced by**: • observations of people's experiences • observations of staff practice • discussions, interviews and surveys with people receiving support, family, friends and visitors • notes of staff, visitors and service user meetings.	Excellent Good Okay Needs more work

✓

S4 Validation: Are people's emotions and feelings recognised, taken seriously and responded to?	How are we doing?
Reflection points: Different people interpret and experience situations and events in different ways. This could be because of past experiences or emotional or physical well-being, as well as the way we think and process information. To provide person-centred care, we have to recognise and respond to what another person is feeling and experiencing. If we don't do this we run the risk of belittling or ignoring someone's feelings, blaming someone or misinterpreting their behaviour. You need to think about the ways in which your organisation's culture impacts upon staff's ability to seek out and validate people's experiences every day. **Consider these statements**: • People's fears and anxieties are always taken seriously and responded to quickly. They are never dismissed or ignored. • Staff understand that someone may interpret what is happening in a different way to others or to how it was intended. They use this knowledge to help them communicate and engage with people. • No one is ever left unattended when they are distressed. If we feel that being alone may help someone to become less distressed, we monitor their well-being throughout. • Our plans for care give staff information about what situations and actions may cause a person distress and how to avoid them. • When someone experiences distress, staff, the person and their family/friends share their knowledge and plan how to prevent distress in the future. • Supporting emotional well-being is considered to be of greater importance than completing practical tasks such as cleaning or tidying. **This can be evidenced by**: • observations of people's experiences • discussions, interviews and surveys with people receiving support and their family, friends and visitors • discussions, interviews and surveys with staff • audits of care plans and daily records with regard to language use.	Excellent Good Okay Needs more work

✓

S5 Enabling: Does the support we provide help people to be as active and involved in their lives as possible? Are people treated as equal partners in their care?	How are we doing?
Reflection points: We can all take for granted the day-to-day decisions we take and things we do for ourselves. The desire to be in control of our own life does not disappear when someone has dementia, but a person may need support to remain involved. In a busy service it is easy for tasks to take over and it can be easy to forget about a person's preferences, skills and desire to be involved. Over time, this can lead to people giving up on the world and retreating into themselves. You need to think about your organisation's culture and how it supports staff to enable people on a daily basis. Person-centred care means involving someone in every aspect of their daily lives and encouraging old and new skills. Treating someone as an equal partner in their care is a more rewarding experience for all. **Consider these statements**: • We always work with someone rather than 'doing to' them. • We encourage people to maintain the skills they have and provide opportunities for them to try new things and develop new skills. • We understand that taking part in normal daily activities can maintain emotional well-being. • Staff demonstrate communication that helps a person to be involved, and they respond to verbal and non-verbal cues from a person. • We understand that the support people will need to take part in any activity may vary on a day-to-day basis. • Choice and options are always given to people in a way that helps them to be involved. **This can be evidenced by**: • observations of people's experiences • discussions, interviews and surveys with people receiving support and their family, friends and visitors • discussions, interviews and surveys with staff • audits of care plans and daily records with regard to use of medication and restraint • records of critical-incident analysis and reflective meetings.	Excellent Good Okay Needs more work

✓

S6 Part of the community: Does our service do all it can to keep people connected with their local community and the local community connected with the service?	How are we doing?
Reflection points: It is easy to take for granted the contact and interaction we have with people and places in our local communities; a trip to the shops, a chat down the pub or just watching the world go by can all be highlights of a day. A person with dementia may need help to maintain these contacts and person-centred care recognises that life extends beyond the 'services' that a person receives. You will need to think about the ways in which your organisation's culture helps a service to seek out and maintain these contacts for people. **Consider these statements**: • There are always visitors coming and going throughout the day and they are helped to take part in the life of our service. • Activities such as going to the local shop, pub, hairdressers or library are all part of everyday life for the people who use our services. • We regularly invite the outside world into the service (through entertainment, events, volunteers etc.). • The routines of our services are flexible so that they do not get in the way of people getting out into the community. • We recognise the importance of nature and animals in improving well-being for people with dementia. • We actively help people to know what is going on in the local community and help them to be involved (organising transport and finding out cinema listings, swimming pool opening times etc.). **This can be evidenced by**: • records and analysis of events and activities in which people participate • audits of availability of community information • discussions, interviews and surveys with people receiving support and their family and friends • audits of outward-facing events.	Excellent Good Okay Needs more work

S7 Relationships: Do we know about, welcome and involve the people who are important to a person?	How are we doing?
Reflection points: Almost everyone has a network of family members and friends, but the onset of dementia can threaten these relationships. By welcoming partners, families and friends into the home, we can support them as well as the person with dementia. If we also help them to understand the dementia journey and how to cope with it, they can become valuable allies for our work. You should think about the ways in which your organisation's culture impacts upon the relationships that are important to people receiving support. **Consider these statements**: • When a person first comes to use our services, we make every effort to find the people who are important to them and help them to be involved. • We welcome anyone who values and loves the person into our service if it is wanted and helpful to the person receiving support. • We know it can be difficult to see a person living with dementia. We share our knowledge and expertise to help friends and family understand what is happening and how to engage with a person. • We understand that supporting the people who are important to a person is a vital part of caring for a person. We provide planned help wherever possible. • The routines of our service are flexible and help people to maintain important relationships (e.g. people can visit whenever they are able). We respect the private space needed for existing relationships. • We do not make assumptions about who may be important in someone's life; instead, we take the lead from the person and what we know about them. We know that important relationships extend beyond 'next of kin' or immediate family. **This can be evidenced by**: • discussions, interviews or surveys with people receiving support and their family, friends and visitors • audits of people's care plans etc. • records of visitor meetings, information days etc. • audits of availability of information regarding how a person can participate in the life of the service.	Excellent Good Okay Needs more work

✓

Points for action	Overall performance on the social environment

✓

References

Alzheimer's Society (2007) *Dementia UK: A Report to the Alzheimer's Society by King's College London and the London School of Economics.* London: Alzheimer's Society.

Alzheimer's Disease International (2010) *World Alzheimer Report 2010: The Global Economic Impact of Dementia.* Available at www.alz.co.uk/research/world-report-2010, accessed on 14 July 2015. London: Alzheimer's Disease International.

Baker, C. J. (2014) *Developing Excellent Care for People Living with Dementia in Care Homes.* London: Jessica Kingsley Publishers.

Bond, J. (2001) 'Sociological Perspectives.' In C. Cantley (ed.) *Handbook of Dementia Care.* Buckingham: Open University Press.

Brod, M., Stewart, A. L., Sands, L. and Walton, P. (1999) 'Conceptualization and measurement of quality of life in dementia.' *The Gerontologist 38,* 25–35.

Brooker, D. (2004) 'What is person-centred care for people with dementia?' *Reviews in Clinical Gerontology 13,* 3, 215–22.

Brooker, D. (2007) *Person Centred Dementia Care: Making Services Better.* London: Jessica Kingsley Publishers.

Brooker, D. (2012) 'Understanding dementia and the person behind the diagnostic label.' *International Journal of Person Centered Medicine 2,* 1, 11–17.

Brooker, D. and Surr, C. (2006) 'Dementia Care Mapping (DCM): Initial validation of DCM 8 in UK field trials.' *International Journal of Geriatric Psychiatry 21,* 1018–25.

Brooker, D. and Surr, C. A. (2016) 'Person-centred Care and Dementia Care Mapping.' In N. A. Pachana (ed.) *Encyclopedia of Geropsychology.* New York, NY: Springer.

Brooker, D. and Woolley, R. (2007) 'Enriching opportunities for people living with dementia: The development of a blueprint for a sustainable activity-based model of care.' *Aging and Mental Health 11,* 4, 371–83.

Brooker, D., Argyle, E., Clancy, D. and Scally, A. (2011) 'Enriched Opportunities Programme: A cluster randomised controlled trial of a new approach to living with dementia and other mental health issues in Extra Care housing schemes and villages.' *Aging and Mental Health 15,* 8, 1008–17.

Brooker, D., La Fontaine, J., De Vries, K. and Latham, I. (2013) 'The development of PIECE-dem: Focussing on the experience of care for people with living with advanced dementia.' *The British Psychological Society Clinical Psychology Forum 250*, October, 38–46.

Brooker, D., La Fontaine, J., Evans, S., Bray, J. and Saad, K. (2014) 'Public health guidance to facilitate timely diagnosis of dementia: ALzheimer's COoperative Valuation in Europe (ALCOVE) Recommendations.' *International Journal of Geriatric Psychiatry 29*, 7, 682–93.

Brooker, D., Latham, I., Evans, S., Jacobson, N., Perry, W., Bray, J., Ballard, C., Fossey, J. and Pickett, J. (2015) 'FITS into practice: Translating research into practice in reducing the use of anti-psychotic medication for people living with dementia in care homes.' *Aging and Mental Health*. DOI: 10.1080/13607863.2015.1063102.

Bryden, C. (2002) 'A person-centred approach to counselling, psychotherapy and rehabilitation of people diagnosed with dementia in the early stages.' *Dementia 1*, 2, 141–56.

Bryden, C. (2005) *Dancing with Dementia: My Story of Living Positively with Dementia.* London: Jessica Kingsley Publishers.

Bryden, C. (2015) *Nothing About Us, Without Us! 20 years of Dementia Advocacy.* London: Jessica Kingsley Publishers.

Chenoweth, L., King, M. T., Jeon, Y-H., Brodaty, H. *et al.* (2009) 'Caring for Aged Dementia Care Resident Study (CADRES) of person-centred care, dementia-care mapping, and usual care in dementia: A cluster-randomised trial.' *The Lancet/Neurology 8*, 317–25.

Cheston, R., Jones, K. and Gilliard, J. (2003) 'Group psychotherapy and people with dementia.' *Aging & Mental Health 7*, 6, 452–461.

Choi, N. G., Ransom, S. and Wyllie, R. (2008) 'Depression in older nursing home residents: The influence of nursing home environmental stressors, coping, and acceptance of group and individual therapy.' *Aging and Mental Health 12*, 5, 536–47.

Clare, L. (2002) 'Developing awareness about awareness in early-stage dementia: the role of psychosocial factors.' *Dementia 1*, 3, 295–312.

Clare, L., Baddeley, A., Moniz-Cook, E. and Woods, R. (2003) 'A quiet revolution.' *The Psychologist 16*, 250–4.

CSCI (Commission for Social Care Inspection) (2008) *See Me, Not Just The Dementia: Understanding Peoples' Experiences of Living in a Care Home.* London: CSCI.

Department of Health (2001) *National Service Framework for Older People.* London: Department of Health.

Department of Health (2010) *Nothing Ventured, Nothing Gained: Risk Guidance for People with Dementia.* London: Department of Health. Available at www.gov.uk/government/uploads/system/uploads/attachment_data/file/215960/dh_121493.pdf, accessed on 14 July 2015.

Deudon, A., Maubourguet, N., Gervais, X., Leone, E. *et al.* (2009) 'Non-pharmacological management of behavioural symptoms in nursing homes.' *International Journal of Geriatric Psychiatry 24*, 12, 1386–95.

Dröes, R. M., Meiland, F. J. M., Lange, J. de, Vernooij-Dassen, M. J. F. J and Tilburg, W. van (2003) 'The meeting centres support programme: An effective way of supporting people with dementia who live at home and their carers.' *Dementia; The International Journal of Social Research and Practice 2*, 3, 426–33.

Edvardsson, D., Sandman, P. O. and Borell, L. (2014) 'Implementing national guidelines for person-centered care of people with dementia in residential aged care: Effects on perceived person-centeredness, staff strain and stress of conscience.' *International Psychogeriatrics 26*, 7, 1171–9.

Eisenhardt, K. and Graebner, M. (2007) 'Theory building from cases: Opportunities and challenges.' *Academy of Management Journal 50*, 1, 25–32.

Feil, N. (1993) *The Validation Breakthrough*. Cleveland: Health Professions Press.

Fossey, J., Ballard, C., Juszczak, E., James, I., Alder, N., Jacoby, R. and Howard, R. (2006) 'Effect of enhanced psychosocial care on antipsychotic use in nursing home residents with severe dementia: A cluster randomised trial.' *British Medical Journal 332*, 756–58.

Francis, R. (2011) The Mid Staffordshire NHS Foundation Trust Public Inquiry Seminar: The role of trust leadership in setting a positive organisational culture. Available at https://www.youtube.com/watch?v=dwnVE4GPbhs, accessed 22 July 2015.

Francis, R. (2013) *Independent Inquiry into Care Provided by Mid Staffordshire NHS Foundation Trust January 2005 – March 2009*. London: TSO.

Frankel, V. (2004) *Man's Search for Meaning* [first published in German in 1946]. London: Rider.

Hawkins, A. H. (2005) 'Epiphanic knowledge and medicine.' *Cambridge Quarterly of Health Economics 14*, 1, 40–60.

Holden, U. P. and Woods, R. T. (1988) *Reality Orientation: Psychological Approaches to the Confused Elderly*. Edinburgh: Churchill Livingstone.

Hughes, J. C. (2001) 'Views of the person with dementia.' *Journal of Medical Ethics 27*, 86–91.

Hughes, J. C. (2011) *Thinking Through Dementia*. Oxford: Oxford University Press.

Hunter, P. V., Hadjistavropoulos, T., Smythe, W. E., Malloy, D. C., Kaasalainen, S. and Williams, J. (2013) 'The Personhood in Dementia Questionnaire (PDQ): Establishing an association between beliefs about personhood and health providers' approaches to person-centred care.' *Journal of Aging Studies 27*, 276–287.

Hunter, P. V, Hadjistavropoulos, T., Smythe, W. E., Malloy, D. C., Kaasalainen, S. and Williams, J. (2013) 'The Personhood in Dementia Questionnaire (PDQ): Establishing an association between beliefs about personhood and health providers' approaches to person-centred care.' *Journal of Aging Studies 27*, 3, 276–87.

Husebo, B. S., Ballard, C., Sandvik, R., Nilsen, O. B. and Aarsland, D. (2011) 'Efficacy of treating pain to reduce behavioural disturbances in residents of nursing homes with dementia: Cluster randomised clinical trial.' *British Medical Journal 343*.

James, I. (2011). *Understanding Behaviour in Dementia That Challenges: A Guide to Assessment and Treatment*. London: Jessica Kingsley Publishers.

Jeon, Y. H., Luscombe, G., Chenoweth, L., Stein-Parbury, J. *et al.* (2012) 'Staff outcomes from the caring for aged dementia care resident study (CADRES): a cluster randomised trial.' *International Journal of Nursing Studies 49*, 5, 508–18.

Killett, A., Burns, D., Kelly, F., Brooker, D. *et al.* (2014) 'Digging deep: How organisational culture affects care home residents' experiences.' *Ageing and Society*. DOI: 10.1017/S0144686X14001299.

Killick, J. and Allan, K. (2001) *Communication and the Care of People with Dementia*. Buckingham: Open University Press.

Killick, J. and Allan, K. (2006) 'The Good Sunset Project: Making contact with those close to death.' *Journal of Dementia Care 14*, 1, 22–24.

Kirkley, C., Bamford, C., Poole, M., Arksey, H., Hughes, J. and Bond, J. (2011) 'The impact of organisational culture on the delivery of person-centred care in services providing respite care and short breaks for people with dementia.' *Health and Social Care in the Community 19*, 4, 438–48.

Kitwood, T. (1987a) 'Dementia and its pathology: In brain, mind or society?' *Free Associations 8*, 81–93.

Kitwood, T. (1987b) 'Explaining senile dementia: The limits of neuropathological research.' *Free Associations 10*, 117–40.

Kitwood, T. (1988) 'The technical, the personal and the framing of dementia.' *Social Behaviour 3*, 161–80.

Kitwood, T. (1989) 'Brain, mind and dementia: With particular reference to Alzheimer's disease.' *Ageing and Society 9*, 1, 1–15.

Kitwood, T. (1990a) 'The dialectics of dementia: With particular reference to Alzheimer's disease.' *Ageing and Society 10*, 177–96.

Kitwood, T. (1990b) 'Understanding senile dementia: A psychobiographical approach.' *Free Associations 19*, 60–76.

Kitwood, T. (1993a) 'Person and process in dementia.' *International Journal of Geriatric Psychiatry 8*, 7, 541–6.

Kitwood, T. (1993b) 'Towards a theory of dementia care: The interpersonal process.' *Ageing and Society 13*, 1, 51–67.

Kitwood, T. (1993c) 'Discover the person, not the disease.' *Journal of Dementia Care 1*, 1, 16–7.

Kitwood, T. (1995a) 'Positive long-term changes in dementia: Some preliminary observations.' *Journal of Mental Health 4*, 2, 133–44.

Kitwood, T. (1995b) 'Building up the mosaic of good practice.' *Journal of Dementia Care 3*, 5, 12–3.

Kitwood, T. (1997a) *Dementia Reconsidered: The Person Comes First*. Buckingham: Open University Press.

Kitwood, T. (1997b) 'The Uniqueness of Persons with Dementia.' In M. Marshall (ed.) *State of the Art in Dementia Care*. London: Centre for Policy on Ageing.

Kitwood, T. (1997c) 'The experience of dementia.' *Ageing and Mental Health 1*, 13–22.

Kitwood, T. and Benson, S. (eds.) (1995) *The New Culture of Dementia Care*. London: Hawker Publications.

Kitwood, T. and Bredin, K. (1992a) *Person to Person: A Guide to the Care of Those with Failing Mental Powers*. Essex: Gale Centre Publications.

Kitwood, T. and Bredin, K. (1992b) 'Towards a theory of dementia care: Personhood and wellbeing.' *Ageing and Society 12*, 269–87.

Lupton, C. and Croft-White, C. (2013) *Respect and Protect: The PANICOA Report*. London: Comic Relief. Available at www.panicoa.org.uk/sites/assets/Final_Main_PANICOA_Report_web.pdf, accessed on 15 July 2015.

May, H., Edwards, P. and Brooker, D. (2009) *Enriched Care Planning for People with Dementia: A Good Practice Guide to Delivering Person-centred Care*. London: Jessica Kingsley Publishers.

McCarthy, B. (2011) *Hearing the Person With Dementia: Person-centred Approaches to Communication for Families and Caregivers*. London: Jessica Kingsley Publishers.

McKeown, J., Clarke, A., Ingleton, C., Ryan, T. and Repper, J. (2010) 'The use of life story work with people with dementia to enhance person-centred care.' *International Journal of Older Peoples Nursing 5*, 2, 148–58.

Morton, I. (1999) *Person-centred Approaches to Dementia Care*. Bicester: Winslow Press Ltd.

NICE/SCIE (National Institute for Health and Clinical Excellence/Social Care Institute for Excellence) (2007) *Dementia: A NICE–SCIE Guideline on Supporting People with Dementia and their Carers in Health and Social Care*. National Clinical Practice Guideline Number 42. London: NICE/SCIE.

Nolan, M., Davies, S. and Grant, G. (2001) *Working with Older People and Their Families: Key Issues in Policy and Practice*. Buckingham: Open University Press.

OECD (2015) *Addressing Dementia: The OECD Response*. Paris: OECD Health Policy Studies, OECD Publishing.

Owen, T. and Meyer, J. (2012) *My Home Life: Promoting Quality Of Life in Care Homes*. York: Joseph Rowntree Foundation.

Packer, T. (1996) 'Shining a light on simple, crucial details.' *Journal of Dementia Care 4*, 6, 22–3.

Passalacqua, S.A. and Harwood, J. (2012) 'VIPS communication skills training for paraprofessional dementia caregivers: An intervention to increase person-centered dementia care.' *Clinical Gerontologist 35*, 5, 425–445.

Perrin, T., May, H. and Milwain, E. (2008) *Wellbeing in Dementia: An Occupational Approach for Therapists and Carers*. 2nd edition. Edinburgh: Churchill Livingstone.

Power, G. A. (2014) *Dementia Beyond Disease: Enhancing Well-being*. Baltimore: Health Professions Press.

Rader, J., Doan, J. and Schwab, M. (1985) 'How to decrease wandering, a form of agenda behaviour.' *Geriatric Nursing 6*, 4, 196–9.

Rogers, C. R. (1961) *On Becoming a Person*. Boston: Houghton Mifflin.

Rokstad, A. M., Røsvik, J., Kirkevold, Ø., Selbaek, G., Benth, J.S. and Engedal, K. (2013) 'The effect of person-centred dementia care to prevent agitation and other neuropsychiatric symptoms and enhance quality of life in nursing home patients: A 10-month randomized controlled trial.' *Dementia Geriatric and Cognitive Disorders 36*, 340–353.

Røsvik, J., Kirkevold, M., Engedal, K., Brooker, D. and Kirkevold, Ø. (2011) 'A model for using the VIPS framework for person-centred care for persons with dementia in nursing homes: A qualitative evaluative study.' *International Journal of Older People Nursing 6*, 227–36.

Røsvik, J., Engedal, K. and Kirkevold, Ø. (2014) 'Factors to make the VIPS Practice Model more effective in the treatment of neuropsychiatric symptoms in nursing home residents with dementia.' *Dementia and Geriatric Cognitive Disorders 37*, 335–346.

Sabat, S. (1994) 'Excess disability and malignant social psychology: A case study in Alzheimer's disease.' *Journal of Community and Applied Psychology 4*, 175–66.

Sabat, S. (2001) *The Experience of Alzheimer's Disease: Life through a Tangled Veil.* Oxford: Blackwell.

Saunderson, H. and Bailey, G. (2013) *Personalisation and Dementia: A Guide for Person-centred Practice.* London: Jessica Kingsley Publishers.

Schein, E. (1990) 'Organizational culture.' *American Psychologist 45*, 2, 109–19.

Smith, S. C., Lamping, D. L., Banerjee, S., Harwood, R. *et al.* (2005) 'Measurement of health-related quality of life for people with dementia: Development of a new instrument (DEMQOL) and an evaluation of current methodology.' *Health Technology Assessment 9*, 10, 1–93, iii–iv.

Stokes, G. (2000) *Challenging Behaviour in Dementia: A Person-centred Approach.* Bicester: Speechmark Publishing.

Stokes, G. and Goudie, F. (1990) *Working with Dementia.* Bicester: Winslow Press.

Thomas, W. H. (1996) *Life Worth Living: How Someone You Love can Still Enjoy Life in a Nursing Home. The Eden Alternative in Action.* Acton, MA: Vanderwyk and Burnam.

Todd, S. J. and Watts, S. C. (2005) 'Staff responses to challenging behaviour shown by people with dementia: An application of an attributional-emotional model of helping behaviour.' *Aging and Mental Health 9*, 1, 71–81.

TSO (2005) *Mental Capacity Act 2005.* London: TSO.

Verity, J. and Kuhn, D. (2008) *The Art of Good Dementia Care: A Guide for Direct Care Staff in Residential Settings.* New York, NY: Thomas Delmar.

Zimbardo, P. (2007) *The Lucifer Effect.* London: Rider.

Subject Index

Author Index